Child-Centred
Nursing

SAGE has been part of the global academic community since 1965, supporting high quality research and learning that transforms society and our understanding of individuals, groups and cultures. SAGE is the independent, innovative, natural home for authors, editors and societies who share our commitment and passion for the social sciences.

Find out more at: **www.sagepublications.com**

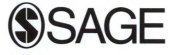

Child-Centred Nursing

Promoting Critical Thinking

Bernie Carter | Lucy Bray | Annette Dickinson

Maria Edwards | Karen Ford

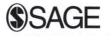

Los Angeles | London | New Delhi
Singapore | Washington DC

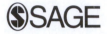

Los Angeles | London | New Delhi
Singapore | Washington DC

SAGE Publications Ltd
1 Oliver's Yard
55 City Road
London EC1Y 1SP

SAGE Publications Inc.
2455 Teller Road
Thousand Oaks, California 91320

SAGE Publications India Pvt Ltd
B 1/I 1 Mohan Cooperative Industrial Area
Mathura Road
New Delhi 110 044

SAGE Publications Asia-Pacific Pte Ltd
3 Church Street
#10-04 Samsung Hub
Singapore 049483

© Bernie Carter, Lucy Bray, Annette Dickinson, Maria Edwards and Karen Ford 2014

First published 2014

Editor: Becky Taylor
Associate Editor: Emma Milman
Production editor: Katie Forsythe
Copyeditor: Rosemary Campbell
Indexer: Caroline Eley
Marketing manager: Tamara Navaratnam
Cover design: Naomi Robinson
Typeset by: C&M Digitals (P) Ltd, Chennai, India
Printed in Great Britain by
CPI Group (UK) Ltd, Croydon, CR0 4YY

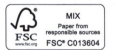

MIX
Paper from responsible sources
FSC www.fsc.org FSC® C013604

Library of Congress Control Number: 2013945922

British Library Cataloguing in Publication data

A catalogue record for this book is available from the British Library

ISBN 978-1-4462-4859-1
ISBN 978-1-4462-4860-7 (pbk)

Contents

About the Authors   ix
Acknowledgements   xi
Publisher's Acknowledgements   xii

**Opening Thoughts: Protecting, Promoting, Sustaining and Enhancing
Children's Potential**   1

What's in a name?   3
Promoting critical thinking   4
Using the book   6
Being passionate and thinking critically   7

1 Approaches to Nursing Children, Young People and their Families   9

Key points   9
Introduction   10
An historical context of children's health care   11
The current context of children's health care   14
Family-centred care   16
   Family-centred care and children and young people with complex needs   18
   Family-centred care: the case for and against   19
   Family-centred care: where to for nursing children and young people?   22
Child-centred care: a further evolution in children's health care   24
   Child-centred care in practice: how are we doing?   27
Transitioning care: another consideration in the care of young people   28
Conclusion   29

**2 Children's and Young People's Position and
Participation in Society, Health Care and Research**   33

Key points   33
Introduction   34
Children and young people: their positioning in society and health care   35
   An historical perspective   36
   The present   37
Children's and young people's participation in health care   39
Children and young people's participation in research   42

Ethical issues   44
Child-centred research approaches   45
Children as participants in research   46
Conclusion   47

3 Consulting and Informing Children and Young People   53

Key points   53
Introduction   54
Gaining and sharing information   54
    Information underpinning interactions   54
    Information about more than the condition   57
Different methods of gaining and sharing information   58
    Consultations and sharing information from health professionals   58
    Written and visual information   61
    Seeking health information from the internet   62
Preparing children and young people for procedures, interventions
    and condition changes   64
    Timing   66
    Content of preparation   67
Conclusion   69

4 Children and Young People Having Choices
   and Making Health Decisions   75

Key points   75
Introduction   76
Making decisions   76
    Making decisions as an adult   76
    Making decisions as a parent   77
    Children and young people making medical decisions   78
Characteristics influencing children and young people's competency   80
    Age   81
    Experience   81
    Presence of parents and family dynamics   82
Involving children and young people in making choices and decisions   86
Children and young people making their own choices   88
The role of children's nurses   91
Conclusion   92

5 How Settings Shape Children's and Young People's Care   97

Key points   97
Introduction   98
The places and spaces of care   98

At home 99
In the community 100
In the hospital 100
In residential care or a long-term care facility 101
Remote care: telemedicine and beyond 103
The impact of health care on child and family space 104
Technology in the home 105
Health professionals and carers 107
Maintaining spaces and places for children and their families 110
Enabling and maintaining family space 110
Affirming the impact 111
Defining the spaces 113
Negotiating and maintaining the boundaries 114
Legal and regulatory influences 115
Conclusion 117

6 Understanding Children's and Young People's Experiences of Illness 121

Key points 121
Introduction 122
Children's and young people's understanding of illness 122
Experiences of being ill 124
Being ill: acute illness 125
Being ill: having cancer 126
Being ill: chronic illness and complex and/or continuing care needs 127
Being in hospital 129
Perceptions of treatment and symptoms 132
Undergoing treatment 132
Experiencing symptoms 135
Fear 136
Fatigue 137
Pain 137
Conclusion 140

7 Examining Practice: Improving the Care of Children and Young People 149

Key points 149
Introduction 150
What is best practice? 150
The scientific view: evidence based nursing 151
The government and organisational view 153
The professional view 153
The consumer view: children's and families' views 154
How do we know when practice is not 'the best'? 155
Changing practice 157

A climate for change   157
A plan for change   159
Responding to change   160
Creating and maintaining a culture of best practice   163
Conclusion   166

Closing Thoughts: Celebrating Success and Aspiring for Better   171

Index   175

About the Authors

Bernie Carter is Professor of Children's Nursing at the University of Central Lancashire and Alder Hey Children's NHS Foundation Trust in the United Kingdom. Her research focuses on children with complex health care needs and life limiting/threatening illness. Bernie is particularly interested in children's experience of symptoms – especially their experience of pain – and how they incorporate the disruptions of illness and disability into their lives. She is the Editor-in-Chief for the *Journal of Child Health Care*.

Lucy Bray is a Reader in Children, Young People and Families at Edge Hill University and Alder Hey Children's NHS Foundation Trust in the United Kingdom. Her research is focused on how children, young people and their parents are prepared, informed and involved in making decisions for planned interventions such as surgery and clinical procedures. She is also interested in how children and young people experience and live day to day with long-term conditions.

Annette Dickinson is a Senior Lecturer and Programme leader for the Post Graduate Child Health Programs at AUT University in New Zealand. She has researched and published in the area of chronic illness/disability in childhood, child and family experiences of health service delivery and nursing practice.

Maria Edwards is a Research Sister at the Clinical Research Facility, Sheffield Teaching Hospitals NHS Foundation Trust in the United Kingdom. She has undertaken both academic and clinical research. Academically Maria's research has focused on children's experiences of being in hospital and their perceptions on being ill and undergoing treatment. Maria also has an interest in children's and families' perspectives of service provision, both hospital and community based.

Karen Ford is Assistant Director of Nursing – Research and Practice Development at the Royal Hobart Hospital, part of the Tasmanian Health Organisation South in Australia. She is also Senior Clinical Lecturer with the School of Nursing and Midwifery, University of Tasmania. Karen's research interests focus on the patient experience and how person-centred approaches can inform and transform healthcare. Children's experiences and care that is centred around the child and family are central concerns in her work.

Acknowledgements

We have had the privilege to meet, care for and work with and share the lives and experiences of many children, young people and families. These experiences have shaped and continue to inspire our lives and work. This book is for all the children, young people and families for whom nurses are part of their lives.

Bernie Carter: For my students, past and present, who inspire me and keep me on my toes.

Lucy Bray: For my parents, Barbara and Trevor, with love always.

Annette Dickinson: To my friends and colleagues at AUT University and Starship Children's Hospital.

Maria Edwards: For Mum and Dad with love. And for John.

Karen Ford: For my parents, Pat and Ron, and for Ross, Paddy, Annie and Will.

Publisher's Acknowledgements

Figure 1.1: The Verandah, Children's Hospital circa 1910, is reproduced with the kind permission of the W.L. Crowther Library, Tasmanian Archive and Heritage Office.

Figure 1.2: Image of contemporary design for a children's ward, is reproduced with kind permission of Alder Hey NHS Trust, Liverpool, UK.

Figure 1.4: Practice development exercise considering family- and child-centred practice is reproduced with kind permission of the Royal Hobart Hospital.

Figure 5.1: Architectural sketch of the Hospital in the Park, Alder Hey Children's NHSFT, is reproduced with kind permission of Alder Hey NSHFT.

Figure 5.2: Children receiving care at Wilson Home, a long term care facility in Auckland, New Zealand (circa 1943) is reproduced with permission of the Alexander Turnbull Library.

Figure 7.1: The Audit Cycle (Benjamin 2008), is reproduced with kind permission of the *British Medical Journal*.

Table 7.1: is republished with permission from the Joanna Briggs Institute.

The following children's drawings in the book are reproduced with kind permission:

Figure I.1, Figure I.2, Figure 3.1, Figure 6.1 and CT.1.

Opening Thoughts: Protecting, Promoting, Sustaining and Enhancing Children's Potential

> Children are our future, numbering over 2.2 billion worldwide (aged 0–19) and representing boundless potential. (World Health Organization 2010: 1)

Nurses who care for, support, advocate, educate, collaborate with and comfort children and young people know that children are our future. Children and young people are at the centre of what we do, how we think and how we act. Nurses working with children and young people aim to promote their health, sustain their well-being, prevent ill health and provide compassionate care when

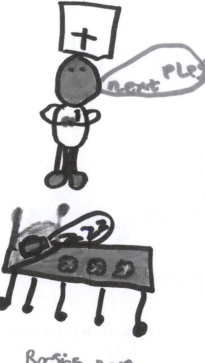

Figure I.1   Rosie's ners (nurse)

they are sick or injured. Regardless of where these nurses are working – in acute, primary or tertiary settings, in the child's home or school – their aim is to support children's boundless potential.

Nurses who work with children and young people see that boundless potential in each and every child they care for. They see that potential in the pre-term baby who requires highly specialised intensive care. They see that potential in the child attending for a routine immunisation. They see that potential in the child coming into hospital for the first, third or thirtieth time. They see that potential in the child whose cognitive impairment is so profound that communication takes exquisitely sensitive attention. They see that potential in the children they care for who are frightened, anxious, distressed, withdrawn, marginalised or disadvantaged. They see that potential in the young person who is achieving independence in their self-care as well as in the adolescent whose illness is robbing them of theirs. They see potential in the situation of a child who is receiving end-of-life care. Although not every child will reach their full potential, nursing care can make a difference to the lives of children and their families.

Nurses who work with children and young people know that children individually and collectively make an important and unique contribution not only to their families but also to the community and society to which they belong. Nurses aim to use their skills, knowledge and understanding in ways that respond in a flexible, informed and individualised way to each child's, young person's and family's

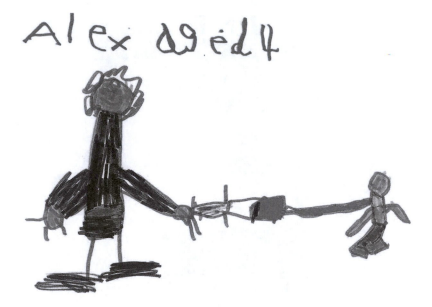

Figure I.2   Alex's drawing of having a blood transfusion (his nurse is the figure on the left)

needs, strengths, hopes and aspirations. Nursing children, young people and their families is no simple task. It is challenging, complex and rewarding but it is not work that we do alone. Nurses work in partnership with children and families. Their work crosses boundaries between disciplines and agencies, between the private world of the home and the more public domain of the hospital. Nursing practice involves understanding how nursing professionals fit into the relational web of children's family ties.

Alongside the technical skills required to deliver high quality care, nursing practice needs to be characterised by being attuned, relational, dialogic, reflexive and committed to understanding the child (Carter et al. 2009). Coming to 'know' a child or young person involves understanding how they are making sense of their illness and trying to determine how the child's life-world is being changed and what these changes will mean for the child. This involves nurses being open to each individual child and, wherever possible, following the child's lead and aligning their care to what has the best resonance for the child. Nurses need to come to know and care for children and young people with 'all our senses' (Stein 2003: 29). Children navigate their worlds with remarkable skill and dexterity, but illness and injury can challenge them. One of the roles of nurses working with children is to offer guidance and support through unfamiliar territory (Carter et al. 2009). Nursing children requires commitment to being child-centred and being willing to take opportunities to provide expert care at all times including those opportunities that arise in the micro-moments of practice.

What's in a name?

While there is generally strong consensus globally that children (from birth to below the age of 18 years) deserve and have the right to be cared for by nurses who have undertaken specific educational preparation to gain specialist skills, knowledge and attributes, there is some dissonance about exactly what these nurses should be called. The key difference lies in whether nurses working with children and young people should be called children's nurses or paediatric nurses. When the five of us started to write this book we knew that we were all professionals with a deep regard for children and a passionate commitment to nursing children, young people and their families. We understood that despite our geographical distance, our different experiences as nurses and our different career trajectories we shared the same values and professional understandings about what made us and our fellow nurses 'tick'. The only real challenge to our consensus was the label we should give ourselves: children's nurses or paediatric nurses. In the United Kingdom (UK) nurses caring for children fought long and hard to move away from the term paediatric nurse as it was felt it resonated too closely with the medical model and the term children's nurse is used by the professional regulation body (Nursing and Midwifery Council 2010). In Australia and New Zealand, the challenge has been different, and the challenge has been to gain recognition of the need for specialist nurses to work with children, so the term paediatric nurse was helpful in this respect. The New Zealand Nurses Organisation talks of nurses who work with children and infants, although within the hospital setting the term 'paediatric nurse' is commonly used, while nurses working in the community often prefer 'child health nurse' as a way of distinguishing their less specialist and more primary health focus. Similarly in Australia, 'paediatric nurse' most often referred to nurses working in acute hospital environments. In recognition that nurses work with children in many different environments, the professional organisations (Australian College of Children's and Young People's Nurses and Council of Children's Nurses) have moved to refer to 'Children's and Young People's Nurses', reflecting the diversity of settings in which the nursing of children takes place. The World Health Organization (2003: 6) opts for 'simplicity' and talks of Children's Nursing while recognising that a variety of terms can be used. We have recognised this tension, which is why we sometimes use the term 'nurses working with children and young people'. Children do not worry about the distinction, they call us nurse; ultimately, the term is less important than the work we do, the values we cherish and the care we deliver.

Promoting critical thinking

In writing this book we have come to know more about nursing children, more about who we are as people who nurse children and who undertake many other roles including practice development, education, research, management, coaching, mentoring, supervision, lobbying and advocacy. We have shared our thoughts, challenged each others' thinking and our own professional, cultural and personal assumptions. Each of us has grown in our understanding of what constitutes best practice in nursing children, young people and their families. The book aims to promote critical thinking and, indeed, it provoked, prompted and powered our own critical thinking.

We believe that nurses working with children, young people and their families need to be critical thinkers as this will help ensure that they consider and then deliver the best possible care. There are many different definitions of critical thinking. Black (2012: 57) notes that 'critical thinking is the analytical thinking which underlies all rational discourse and enquiry. It is characterized by a meticulous and rigorous approach'. Borglin (2012: 612), talking about nurse education, summarises critical thinking as being 'characterised by logical and consistent thinking, a controlled sense of scepticism or disbelief about assertions and conclusions, taking stock of existing information while identifying holes and weaknesses and, finally, freedom from bias and prejudice'. The concepts underpinning critical thinking are important. Children and their families deserve care which is underpinned by the best evidence and delivered by knowledgeable nurses who are able

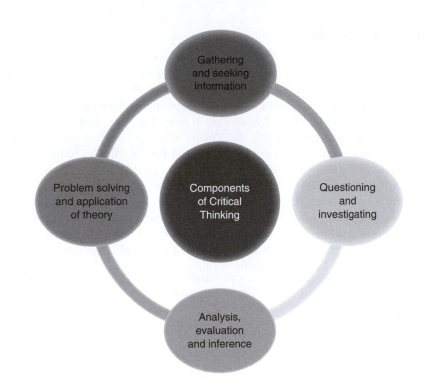

Figure I.3   Four key components of critical thinking (developed from Chan 2013)

to challenge and refine practice. Although there are many different models, Chan (2013) notes that critical thinking within nursing is composed of four main components (see Figure I.3).

Critical thinking could just be an 'armchair' or desk-based activity, limited to thinking *about* practice but never translating the outcomes of thinking into the myriad of different situations and challenges that are posed within practice settings. Nursing children and young people requires much of nurses; it is complex work that requires nurses to think *and* do. Connected to critical thinking is the notion of 'fluid intelligence' which reflects an ability 'to determine patterns, make connections and solve new problems' (Ordonez 2012: 3). Best practice arises from when we attend carefully to the needs, views and perspectives of the children we care for and align our critical thinking skills and our fluid intelligence along with a compassionate approach to our care. Compassion has recently been described as 'intelligent kindness' (Commissioning Board Chief Nursing Officer and DH Chief Nursing Adviser 2012: 13), which is an attractive term to sum up what is central to nursing children and young people.

Using the book

This book focuses on the core principles that underpin practice and it focuses on the broad theories and concepts that inform and shape the practice of nurses working with children and young people. In the seven main chapters we explore children's positioning in society and how that frames the way they are involved in health care and decision making. We examine family-centred care and child-centred care and we consider our past, contemporary and future roles as nurses in delivering care. We explore children's right to participate, be informed and make choices about their health and lives. We examine the places and spaces of care and the ways in which technology creates new opportunities and constraints on children's lives. We consider how children and young people experience illness and how we, as nurses, can help make these experiences meaningful, mitigate potential trauma and promote well-being. We also consider what constitutes best practice and how we are responsible for helping to achieve this.

Case Studies

We have woven case studies throughout the chapters as a means of helping translate the concepts and theories into the world of practice. We see these as starting points for your thinking about how the theory and concepts can guide, inform and shape practice.

In Chapter 1 you meet Mikael (aged 4), his parents (Catherine and John) and his siblings (Sam aged 6; Sarah aged 1). Mikael has just been diagnosed with Type 1 diabetes mellitus. This case study follows Mikael's initial diagnosis and care as well as the support and education he and his family receive about managing his diabetes.

In Chapter 2 you meet Danny (aged 15 years) who, soon after his 15th birthday, was diagnosed with Hodgkins lymphoma. This case study explores Danny's response to treatment, his resistance to hospitalisation and how his care team created an alternative pathway for his chemotherapy and follow-up management.

In Chapter 3 you meet Jayden (aged 8 years), his mother (Alison) and his grandma. Jayden is being investigated for suspected appendicitis. Much of the focus of this case study is on the issues around informing and preparing Jayden for having an intravenous cannula inserted.

In Chapter 4 you meet Rachel (aged 14 years) who has lived with a long-term continence condition since she was born. This case study explores some of the tensions that can develop as a young person's self-care choices and decisions come into conflict with those of her parents.

In Chapter 5 you meet Sarah (aged 12 years), her brother Frankie (aged 9) who has complex health care needs, her parents and Frankie's caregiver (Simon). This case study explores Sarah's experiences of Frankie's care needs and the impact of having carers in her family home.

In Chapter 6 you meet Harry (aged 5 years) and his mother. This case study explores Harry's fears and concerns as he thinks about having to go to the hospital to have his tonsils removed; it also explores his experiences of being in hospital.

In Chapter 7 you meet Beth, a nurse trying to implement change within a hospital. This case study explores some of the individual, organizational and other challenges that Beth faced in planning, implementing and evaluating change.

TED Boxes

Since the mission of the book is to 'promote critical thinking' we have developed critical thinking TED activities. These TED activities require you to Think, Explore and evaluate, and Decide and discuss (see box below). We have provided a range of prompts and suggested activities to help the theories and concepts we discuss become more real as you relate these to situations and settings you have and are experiencing, and the children, young people and families you are caring for.

T	hink about whether aspects of your practice are underpinned by any beliefs, traditions or ways of working that may not be based on evidence.
E	xplore and evaluate the evidence, perspectives and strategies you have read in the literature and in policy and other documents.
D	ecide, based on your reflections, how you could improve your practice. Discuss your findings with your colleagues.

Being passionate and thinking critically

The New Zealand Nurses Organisation (2013: 1) states that 'all children, at some point in their lives, will come into contact with nurses'. We passionately believe that when children do come into contact with a nurse they should receive care that is skilled and takes account of each child's particular needs and circumstances, and that the outcome of the care they receive is the best it possibly can be. When we do this, we know it can make a positive difference to children's and their families' lives. Josie, aged 10 years, knows that nurses are important.

When I was little, about two years ago I got sick. I was at school and got a very sick stomach. It hurt a lot, a lot more even than the time my brother had kicked me instead of the football. I went to hospital and they gave me some medicine and the pain went away. I said to mum 'Let's go home now' but the doctor said my stomach was sick and I needed an operation to make it better. I didn't want an operation. I told my mum 'I want to go home NOW!' Mum said I had to have the operation and then she cried. Dad didn't cry but he sounded a bit funny. My nurse was Paula and she talked to me. She said everyone in the hospital wanted me to get better but I couldn't get better if I went home. She said she was in charge of making sure I got better. I said I was frightened of hospital. Paula talked to me and explained things to me and she held my hand and she made me giggle. Paula helped me a lot, she made me smile when I was scared and made me feel safe when I was in the hospital. She was a good nurse.

We hope that this book equips and inspires you to become passionate, critical thinking, 'good' nurses who will help make a difference to children, young people and families. We believe that nurses who care for children and young people have boundless potential to make these differences.

References

Black, B. (2012) *A to Z of Critical Thinking*. London: Continuum International Publishing.

Borglin, G. (2012) 'Promoting critical thinking and academic writing skills in nurse education', *Nurse Education Today*, 32(5): 611–613.

Carter, B., Marshall, M. and Sanders, C. (2009) 'An exquisite knowing of children', in R.C. Locsin and M. Purnell (eds) *Contemporary Process of Nursing: The (Un)Bearable Weight of Knowing Persons in Nursing*. New York: Springer Publishing.

Chan, Z.C.Y. (2013) 'A systematic review of critical thinking in nursing education', *Nurse Education Today*, 33(3): 236–240.

Commissioning Board Chief Nursing Officer and DH Chief Nursing Adviser (2012) *Compassion in Practice*. Department of Health, NHS Commissioning Board, www.commissioningboard.nhs.uk

New Zealand Nurses Organisation (2013) *Nurses Working with Children and Infants*. Wellington: New Zealand Nurses Organisation.

Nursing and Midwifery Council (2010) *Children's Nurses*. Available at: www.nmc-uk.org/Get-involved/Consultations/Past-consultations/By-year/Pre-registration-nursing-education-Phase-2/What-do-nurses-do/Childrens-nurses/ (accessed 9 October 2013).

Ordonez, K. (2012) *Critical Thinking and Its Applications*. Delhi: Orange Apple.

Stein, H.F. (2003) 'Ways of knowing in medicine: seeing and beyond', *Families, Systems & Health: The Journal of Collaborative Family Health Care*, 21(1): 29–35.

World Health Organization (2003) *WHO Europe Children's Nursing Curriculum. WHO European Strategy for Continuing Education for Nurses and Midwives*. Geneva: World Health Organization.

World Health Organization (2010) *Global Recommendations on Physical Activity for Health*. Geneva: World Health Organization.

Chapter 1

Approaches to Nursing Children, Young People and their Families

Key points

- Caring for children, young people and their families requires well developed understandings of the health, psychological, developmental, communication and cultural needs of each child and young person.
- The family is an integral part of how children and young people experience and engage in society and health care.
- Family-centred care and child-centred care are key philosophies underpinning the nursing care of children and young people; however, their application in practice is not without problems.
- Children are not a homogenous group and each child has their own individual perspectives and experiences.
- Children and young people with complex care needs require special considerations to ensure their health, well-being and rights are met.
- Transitioning from paediatric to adult care settings can present issues for young people, their parents and health care professionals.

Key theories and concepts explored in this chapter are child-centred care, family-centred care, children participating in their care and transitioning between services.

Case study 1.1: Mikael

Setting the scene

Mikael is 4 years old and has just been diagnosed with type 1 diabetes mellitus. He lives with his parents, Catherine and John and his two siblings, Sarah aged 1 year and Sam aged 6 years. Mikael is an active, inquisitive child, who is 'into everything'. The

(Continued)

(Continued)

family moved to the area a couple of years ago, so do not have an extended family support network close by.

Mikael was admitted to hospital in diabetic ketoacidosis and spent two days in intensive care for initial stabilisation. He was then transferred to the children's ward for further care and education. He spent a total of six days in hospital. The time Mikael was in intensive care was a very stressful time for the family and they also needed to come to terms with Mikael's unexpected and new diagnosis of type 1 diabetes. Because of his young age, Mikael will be fully reliant on his parents for the monitoring and management of his diabetes, including initially six finger pricks a day to monitor blood glucose levels, insulin injections morning and evening, his diet and general well-being.

John (Mikael's father) needed to return to work after the first three days of Mikael's hospitalisation. He travels across town to his job and works long hours. This meant that Mikael's mother, Catherine, was taught the skills she needed to be able to care for Mikael and she was expected to teach John these skills. Catherine stayed with Mikael for the first two nights on the children's ward but was not able to stay for the other nights. The family only had one car and so on the last two days of his admission, Catherine and the baby travelled an hour to the hospital by bus after seeing Sam off to school. Although Catherine missed being there for Mikael's morning insulin on these days, she was there during the day to receive education and for his evening dose of insulin. John called in to spend a short but enjoyable time with Mikael before taking Catherine and the baby home, and picking Sam up from a friend's place along the way.

Introduction

This chapter focuses on the philosophical underpinnings of children's and young peoples' nursing. In the discussion that follows you will be encouraged to reflect on the philosophies of family- and child-centred care, what they mean to you in your practice, the points of tension and challenges that exist, and the care of children, young people and their families more generally. The case study provides a means for reflection on how children and families experience health care and what informs ways of working with them. This includes some of the taken-for-granted aspects of care and also best practice and possibilities for achieving child- and family-centred care.

A number of assumptions underpin the discussion throughout the chapter. Firstly, children and young people experience illness, injury and disability in a different way from adults and their health care needs are therefore quite different to those of adults. Further, children's and young people's developmental immaturity leads to certain vulnerabilities. Their vulnerability is not an inherent consequence of childhood or adolescence as such, but a result of adult-centric social structures and services that children and young people cannot access as easily as adults. In addition, childhood and adolescence are characterised by rapid physical, cognitive, developmental, social and experiential changes. Children's and young people's dependence on adults is naturally on a continuum of dependence to growing independence – although this latter point may not necessarily be the case for children with long-term complex conditions (Children's Hospitals Australasia 2010). Care of

children and young people also involves unique considerations in terms of communication, consent (or assent) and confidentiality (Ford et al. 2007).

Societal and economic impacts provide varying contexts for children's lives in the
21st century. For example, women's increased participation in the workforce and
changes to family structures (including the increased numbers of single parent families and of childless families) impact on children within families and in the broader
society. Intergenerational relationships also need consideration, particularly with the
increasing numbers of frail older people requiring care and support within families
and society (Christensen and Prout 2005: 51).

Children and young people experience health care services in many different settings, such as in their homes, their community and in hospital settings. While much of
the literature relates to the care of children in hospital, it must be acknowledged that
health care for children largely takes place outside of hospital wards and clinics. Caring for children with complex needs within the home, for example, poses different and
sometimes quite complex issues about how health care professionals work in family-
centred ways (Kuo et al. 2012).

A further important assumption for nursing children and young people is that
nurses who provide this care need to have well-developed skills to recognise the
particular health, psychological, emotional, developmental, communication and cultural needs of each child and young person (Hill et al. 2011: 80).

An historical context of children's health care

Tracing the historical place in which children and young people have been positioned in health care, whether that care is within the community or in hospital,
shows that it has been largely influenced by their positioning within society
more generally. The roles families play in their child's health care have also been
impacted by social drivers. Advances in preventative health such as the impact
of immunisation as well as treatments and technology, policies and legislation
(most notably of course in affluent societies) have also shaped how and where
children and young people are cared for. Once fatal childhood diseases such as
congenital heart defects or leukaemia are now treatable, and many children in
countries with appropriate resources can now survive into adulthood (Stang and
Joshi 2006).

When considering the history of the care of children in hospital, the 19th and
earlier part of the 20th centuries saw parents excluded from the wards and denied
the opportunity to be with their child. The understanding at that time was that children in hospital settled better when parents did not visit. During this same period,
parents of children with severe disabilities were strongly urged to institutionalise
their children, resulting in these 'hopeless cases' being physically removed and separated from their families. The environment considered suitable for the hospital-based
care of children has changed considerably since the first wards built for children.
Figure 1.1 shows a photograph of a children's ward at the beginning of the 20th
century and Figure 1.2 shows architectural drawings of the wards of the 'Hospital in
the Park' in Liverpool, UK, which is due to be completed in autumn 2015. These

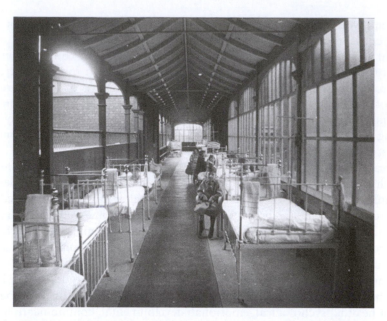

Figure 1.1 The Verandah, Children's Hospital circa 1910. (Image reproduced with the kind permission of the W.L. Crowther Library, Tasmanian Archive and Heritage Office.)

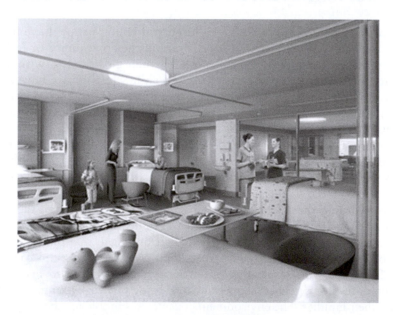

Figure 1.2 Image of contemporary design for a children's ward. (Reproduced with kind permission of Alder Hey NHS Trust, Liverpool, UK.)

starkly contrasting environments reflect very different ways of thinking about what is necessary to be able to deliver good health care to children.

The hospital rules from a children's hospital in 1947 limiting parents visiting their hospitalised children are presented in Figure 1.3. The strict and inflexible rules outlined here appear similar to those for visiting prison inmates (Street 1992). While the regulations and practices intended to safeguard the best interests of the ill child, such practices did not support the interests of the parent or child so much as institutional interests (Street 1992). For example, medical staff determined how often, and for how long, children might be with their parents.

The strong emotional reactions of children to their parents when they were allowed to visit was seen as evidence that parental visits had a detrimental effect on children's well-being. The recognition that the practice of separating children and parents could cause possible psychological trauma to children who experienced hospitalisation was slow to develop. Following on from societal reactions to the effects World War II had on the separation of children from their families, the subsequent work of people such as child psychologists John Bowlby and James and Joyce Robertson on separation, and reports such as the Platt Report (Ministry of Health 1959), children's health care in the second half of the 20th century saw changes in care practices. As a result, the involvement of parents in the care of their sick child became an accepted feature of children's nursing. In Australia, daily visiting for children was adopted in the 1950s and 1960s and mothers whose young babies were sick were able to be with their children in hospital in the late 1970s (Wood 2008: 123). Sibling visits and parents accompanying their children to theatre were other changes to care practices around this time (Kuo et al. 2012). However, the recognition that the interests of children, young people and families should be at the centre of children's health care was slow to pervade all areas of children's health care.

Patients are not allowed visitors unless they have been in the hospital for a period of four weeks, after which time only the parents or guardians (no friends or relatives are allowed) are permitted to visit on each alternate Sunday in each month, between the hours of 2 p.m. and 3.30 p.m. Parents or guardians of patients dangerously ill are allowed to visit as often as the Doctors consider necessary.

Parents or guardians of patients in the Baby Wards and Infectious Wards are only allowed to visit with the special permission of the Medical Superintendent or his Deputy.

These regulations apply to the hospital section ... and have been made to protect the interests of the patients in the Hospital...

Lollies, Cakes, Biscuits, etc., must not be brought to the Hospital for patients. Raw or dried fruits, nuts, eggs and nourishing foods are of benefit, but must be handed to the Sister of the Ward. (Royal Children's Hospital)

Figure 1.3 Hospital visiting rules 1947 (cited in Street 1992: 11)

The description by Joy Chester – founder of AWCH (the (Australian) Association for the Wellbeing of Children in Healthcare), of her experiences around the admission to hospital of her child illustrates this:

> In July, 1969, my 6 year old son was hospitalised at a major children's hospital in Sydney. I stayed with him for four days. The ward TV-set proudly showed man taking his first steps on the moon, while below it, lonely babies and children cried, rocked or were quietly withdrawn. The contrast of advanced scientific technology and the neglect of the emotional needs of those children was overwhelming. (cited in Wood 2008: 124)

The current context of children's health care

Despite significant progress and initiatives to address the negative experiences of children who are hospitalised, children continue to experience physical harm, unnecessary pain, fear and anxiety during and after health care experiences (Nicholson and Clarke 2007). A number of reports and inquiries have highlighted continuing deficits in health care services where bureaucratic and systemic interests have been privileged over those of children and young people. In the UK, for example, the Bristol Inquiry Report was instigated in response to the deaths of some 30 to 35 children undergoing cardiac surgery between 1991 and 1995 that were found to be the result of major 'flaws and failures within the hospital, its organisation and culture' (Kennedy 2001: 154). The report found that in health care services children were treated as 'mini adults', simply needing 'smaller beds and smaller portions of food' and that information was not provided in a suitable form for children or their parents. Further, it was reported that staff did not have specific education in caring for children and that the facilities did not meet the special needs of young children, older children, adolescents or parents (Kennedy 2001: 12). The Garling Report (2008) was conducted in the Australian state of New South Wales and included a review of health care services for children and young people following adverse events that shocked the public, including the death of a young person whose care was found to be inadequate. These reports and others have led to significant policy and practice changes that emphasise the importance of placing children, young people and families at the centre of care. Many policies that have been developed for the standards and rights of children's and young people's health care are framed by the United Nations Convention on the Rights of the Child (UN 1989) that encapsulates the universal rights of children.

The UN Convention on the Rights of the Child (UNCRC) was adopted by the United Nations General Assembly in 1989. It acknowledges the status, role and rights of children and their needs and situations by setting standards in health care, education and legal and social services (UN 1989). Articles of the Convention that directly relate to health care are outlined in Table 1.1. National and international standards for health care aim to achieve child-centred health services and are underpinned and

Table 1.1   Articles of the UN Convention on the Rights of the Child that relate directly to children's health care (Nicholson and Clarke 2007)

Article	As the Article relates to health care
2	Equal rights to care with no discrimination for any reason
3	Whenever an adult makes any decision about a child or takes any action that affects the child this should be what is best for the child
6	The right to live
7	The right to name and nationality, and to be cared for by parents
9	The right to remain with parents, or in contact with parents, unless this is contrary to the child's 'best interests'
12 and 13	The right to receive information and express views and ideas freely
19	The right to be protected from any form of harm, including violence, neglect and all types of abuse
23	The right of those with a disability (physical or mental) to lead a full and decent life within their community
24	The right to the highest standard of health and medical care attainable
27	The right to a standard of living adequate for physical, mental, spiritual, moral and social development
28	The right to education
30	The right of a child belonging to an ethnic, religious or linguistic minority to enjoy their culture, practise their religion and use their language
31	The right to rest and play
38	The right to be protected from and during armed conflicts, and not to be recruited to take part in hostilities, especially before the age of 15 years
42	Is about the duty of the state to ensure that children's rights relating to health are made known

informed by the UNCRC. As an example, the World Health Organization's Child Friendly Healthcare Initiative (Southall et al. 2000) aims to achieve internationally applicable standards for practices in hospitals and health centres. The health care standards proposed in the initiative are based on children's rights as expressed in the UNCRC.

The Australian National Standards for Children and Adolescents in Health Care (RACP 2008) also reflect the rights of children as outlined in the UNCRC and aim to ensure quality care for children and young people in an environment that is 'safe and appropriate for the age and stage of development of the child or adolescent' (RACP 2008: 3). In addition, these standards recognise the special health care needs of children and young people; that they need to be cared for by specially trained staff; and that children require separate facilities in all areas of the health care service where they are cared for (RACP 2008). The European Association for Children in Hospital (EACH) is another example of an organisation concerned with children's health care. EACH is the umbrella organisation for 13 national associations in Europe involved in the welfare of all children before, during or after a stay in hospital. EACH was established to promote the implementation of the European Charter for Children in Hospital and the 10 principles of the EACH Charter relate in many respects to the rights of the child as outlined in the UNCRC.

As a result of such initiatives, children's contemporary experiences of health care are different in many ways to those of earlier times. These changes manifest the rights of children as outlined in the UNCRC (UN 1989). For example, the child's right to remain with their parents is expressed in Article 9 of the Convention, and one important feature in contemporary children's health care is increased parental presence and support. Hospital rules that once limited parental visits have (although we would argue – not universally) been replaced with policies that support parents residing in hospital.

Family-centred care

> When I got to hospital it was good to have dad there. Mum had to stay home and look after my big brother. (11-year-old boy, Ford 2010)

The case for working *with* children, young people and their families is now recognised as fundamental to the care of children and young people. Children are dependent on their families in all aspects of their daily lives and it is the context of family that is most instrumental to children's and young people's growth and development (Children's Hospitals Australasia 2010). It makes sense that the nursing care of children, young people and their families places their interests at the centre of their care. Family-centred care (FCC) is the most common philosophical approach underpinning health care delivery for children and young people in Western countries such as the UK, Australia, New Zealand, the United States and Canada. Since its inception FCC has had various forms and its definitions have evolved with time. However, in essence FCC is a way of working in partnership with a family. Essentially FCC recognises that children need to be cared for in the context of their family and that the family is both the constant in a child's life and should be central in the child's plan of care (Ahmann 1994). The philosophy of FCC, in effect, intends a more equal partnership between the health professional and parent in the health care of the child. Principles of FCC (based on those developed by American organisations including Family Voices and the Institute for Family- and Patient-Centred Care) are presented in the Table 1.2.

The more recent definition of FCC by Shields et al. (2006) recognises all the family members as care recipients, because when a child is admitted to hospital, the whole family is affected. FCC should inform the health care of children in their homes and in other community settings. Shields et al. (2006) describes FCC as a way of caring for children and their families within health services that ensures care is planned around the

Table 1.2   General principles of family-centred care (adapted from Kuo et al. 2012: 298)

Information sharing	The exchange of information is open, objective and unbiased
Respect and honouring differences	The working relationship is marked by respect for diversity, cultural and linguistic traditions, and care preferences
Partnership and collaboration	Appropriate decisions that best fit the health care needs, strengths, values and abilities of all involved are made together by involved parties, including families, at the level they choose
Negotiation	The desired outcomes of care plans are flexible and not necessarily absolute
Care in the context of family and community	Direct health care and decision making reflect the child within the context of his/her family, home, school, daily activities and quality of life within the community

whole family, not just the individual child/person. A family-centred approach to children's and young people's health care recognises that their emotional and developmental needs as well as overall family well-being are best achieved when the system supports the abilities and choices of the family to meet the needs of their child (Shields et al. 2008).

Family structures in Western societies are increasingly complex and dynamic. Families can include blended families, single-parent households, adoptive homes, same-sex couples, and members of the extended family. A family-centred approach recognises diversity among families including family structures, backgrounds, goals, strategies, actions and strengths. It includes respect for personal and cultural beliefs and the importance of incorporating these beliefs into health care choices. Such an approach also recognises that families experience differences in family support and service delivery and have different information needs.

Case study 1.2: Mikael

Planning and caring for all the family

Care for Mikael's diabetes must involve his family as it will have impacts on all family members such as influencing their food choices and the timing of family meals. Mikael's family was advised that they should all eat together and have the same foods, rather than preparing 'special' food for Mikael. The Diabetes Nurse Educator (DNE) knows that, as the family learns to manage and to live with Mikael's diabetes, there will be a strong focus on this new aspect of his life and theirs.

Catherine cares for the children during the week and John is the primary carer at the weekends when Catherine is at work. This employment pattern reflects shifts in family structures and functions in Western society which means that fathers may not be the

(Continued)

(Continued)

sole 'breadwinner' in a family and parents often share direct parenting responsibilities. John needs to be able to manage Mikael's care at the weekends, including giving him his morning insulin and preparing meals.

When providing Catherine's education, the DNE assessed Catherine's confidence and skills in being able to manage Mikael's diabetes regime and used a number of supports to help her, including written material, experience in administering insulin to Mikael with supervision as well as using skin models to practise on. They also talked about the different 'diabetes scenarios' that might occur and how these could be managed. These scenarios included what to do if Mikael's blood sugar drops too low, what to do if the insulin vial is dropped on the floor or what to do when Mikael has a 'sick day' (is unwell). The DNE also worked to ensure Catherine could teach these skills to John.

The DNE encouraged Mikael to participate in his care as much as possible, by giving consideration to his individual development and abilities. Although he protested about the needles, his parents were advised to take a positive approach to Mikael's involvement and the treatment. So they encouraged him to be involved by washing his hands, doing his finger pricks and taking part in choosing the injection site. In time, as he became more accepting of the injections, he also pushed the plunger on the syringe.

The DNE was aware from the start of Mikael's care that the inclusion of his siblings also needed consideration. When Mikael was first diagnosed, 6- year-old Sam was frightened that Mikael was very sick in hospital and that he might die. The DNE suggested that Catherine brought Sam to the hospital one afternoon to see and to play with his brother. The visit alleviated his fears and the nurses on the ward provided Sam with age-appropriate information about Mikael, explaining that Mikael had a medical condition and he needed to have special medicine to keep him safe. Mikael and Sam played a game together and Mikael showed Sam how he did his own finger prick and how it did not really hurt.

Family-centred care and children and young people with complex needs

Children are not a homogenous group, and children and young people, such as those with disabilities, those in out-of-home care, those from culturally and linguistically diverse backgrounds and refugees require additional services to address their specific needs (Children's Hospitals Australasia 2010: 6).

Children with complex needs are a broad group of children with very diverse needs, including those children requiring long-term ventilator support, children needing assisted enteral or parenteral nutrition, children requiring administration of intravenous medication, children with mobility or sensory impairment, children with behavioural needs and children with life limiting or life threatening conditions. Increasing survival rates for children with complex conditions and for those born prematurely means that the numbers of children in this group is growing.

Children with complex care needs require increased health services beyond those generally required by healthy children. Frequently their health care needs are inextricably part of their everyday lives and treatments and technologies may overlay and dominate their lives and have a profound impact on other family members such as their siblings. However, despite these differences, many children with complex care needs have the same wishes and needs as other children. Things that matter to them include living at home, going to school, spending time with friends and participating in recreational and community activities with family and peers, and these things are also important to their families (Social Care Institute for Excellence 2008). Woodgate et al. (2012) explored the impact that caring for a child with complex needs has on parents' and families' levels of participation in everyday life. They referred to the notion of 'having a life' which entailed feelings of belonging, of being accepted and being able to contribute to the spaces they participate in. This sense of having a life required access to resources and significant 'physical, mental, psychological and spiritual work' by parents, that was sometimes found to be very difficult to sustain.

Children and young people with complex health needs and their families often require high levels of physiological, psychological and social care that brings them and their families into contact with a wide range of services; health care professionals are but one group among many (Carter et al. 2007). There is a recognised need for a 'seamless web' of care, treatment and support and for real partnerships between health and social care agencies that includes the child or young person and family as integral participants. However, while this seamless web is the ideal, studies demonstrate that families' experience of services is often not seamless (Carter et al. 2007) and they may not be treated as equal members in the partnership because 'experts' exert their power. Yet despite these challenges, many parents of children with complex needs very quickly become the experts in caring for their child and, as previously recognised, they are often expected to act in this role. The notion of how children and young people live with special or complex conditions will be explored in more detail in Chapter 5 of this book.

Family-centred care: the case for and against

While children's nurses generally espouse the philosophy of FCC for all children and families as the ideal approach to care, effective collaboration and the meaningful involvement of families may, in fact, be quite challenging to achieve. FCC is a complex and sophisticated relational dynamic that is influenced by a number of internal and external factors (Carter 2008). The case for and against FCC needs to be considered carefully, as do the possible ways forward.

The case for FCC as a fundamental premise is a strong one. FCC, in its different forms as a way of working and being with families, has been fairly universally embraced by practitioners, educationalists and researchers for more than 50 years (for example, *The Platt Report* in the UK (Ministry of Health 1959) and Australian Paediatric Association (1958, cited in Hill et al. 2011)). This is certainly the case in many so-called 'developed' countries such as UK, USA, New Zealand and Australia, as well as in less well resourced countries. FCC presents a way of approaching caring for children, young people and their families that nurses recognise as important. Nurses also find it a satisfying and rewarding way of working (Carter 2008), and the concept of FCC as an approach for working with families is supported by health care institutions as well as service user groups representing children's and parents' interests (for example AWCH; NAWCH; Institute for Patient- and Family-Centred Care). Yet, tensions exist in the ways that FCC is realised in practice and FCC continues to be inadequately and only partly implemented in clinical practice (Kuo et al. 2012). The complexities and discordances in understanding and expectations of FCC in relation to parent participation have been identified in a number of studies (Coyne and Cowley 2007; Darbyshire 1994; Power and Franck 2008). In addition, there is little evidence around the attainability of FCC as a model for health care delivery.

A systematic review of qualitative studies (Shields et al. 2008) indicated that there was a paucity of evidence around FCC and its effectiveness. FCC was found to be problematic due to the difficulties and barriers such as relational and attitudinal issues that compromise the effectiveness and implementation of FCC – in its fullest sense – in daily practice. It is also recognised that there has been a lack of attention to the skills, support and resources nurses need to enable them to practice in family-centred ways (Barnsteiner et al. 1994: 36). The leadership and culture of an organisation are other factors important to the effective implementation of this model because systemic processes, both overt and implicit, that support the child and family being at the centre are essential. Mikkelsen and Frederiksen's (2011) concept analysis concluded that FCC is only a 'partially mature concept' (p. 1159) and that the 'perspective of the ill child is not very prominent in the current conceptualization of FCC' (p. 1160). As organisations and settings for children's health care change, with a shift from inpatient to ambulatory care, there are additional and new challenges for the provision of FCC.

There is a general recognition that children's admission to hospital should be avoided wherever possible, because of the negative impacts hospitalisation has on children emotionally, psychologically and developmentally, as well as the potential physical risks to them. When a child's admission to hospital is necessary, admission should be for as short a time as possible. The resource costs associated with hospital care, technological advances and economic imperatives have also influenced this shift, so that increasingly out of hospital care is a feature of children's and young people's health care. However, shorter admission times to hospital means that time for the nurse to get to know the child and family can be limited (Ford 2011). Quicker throughput means that time for preparation, finding out about individual family needs and preferences as well as the provision of information about care following discharge are also limited. For example, research around the post-discharge care needs for families (Ford et al. 2012) following the child's admission for surgery has highlighted that while many families receive the information they require to manage care of the child following discharge, this is not always the case. This lack of information then impacts on symptom management, for example the prevention and treatment of pain. An example of one initiative by nurse researchers to provide alternative information sources to improve symptom management after short-stay surgery is the development of online resources with parents for parents (http://www.mychildisinpain.org.uk/).

Even when health professionals believe that family-centred care is a central value within their care practices, families may not always see this as the case. A study of FCC practices within a paediatric intensive care unit in Canada (Mac-Donald et al. 2012) questioned the integration of family-centred care practices into the sociocultural context of a paediatric intensive care setting. Findings indicated that there was a divergence between espoused FCC practices and the lived experiences of family members. The researchers suggest that these structures transform the child into a medicalised object – 'the patient' – and the parents are displaced to being the 'visitor'. While staff made efforts to personalise bed spaces with items such as the child's own toys or photos, these spaces, in fact 'belonged' to staff and parents struggled even to find room to be with their child. Whilst Roets et al. (2012) note that managers need to take responsibility for ensuring the emotional support of parents as part of FCC within the paediatric intensive care setting but equally, all nurses have a responsibility for caring for parents.

We suggest that in considering the role of parents and family, nurses need to reflect on how parents and other family members are positioned. As an example, parents and family members might be referred to as 'visitors' in the hospital setting. Even the use of terms such as 'open visiting' for parents in ward information sheets carries with it connotations about the role parents are allocated. MacDonald et al. (2012) propose that in using such language, family members are relegated to a role that does not recognise their centrality and that when parents are present with their sick child, rather than visiting, parents are in fact *parenting*.

Whilst parents in general want and expect to participate in their child's hospital care, the level of parental involvement may be vexed and contentious. There is evidence that parents in contemporary paediatric settings feel increasingly pressured to participate in their child's care, taking on responsibilities that may traditionally be seen as 'nurses' work' (Coyne and Cowley 2007). Parents are increasingly asked or expected to be involved in more complex responsibilities such as monitoring and coordination roles. This is seen to correspond with an increasing expectation by nurses who take parents' participation for granted (Coyne and Cowley 2007; Shields et al. 2006). However, the increasing expectations placed upon parents have been found to some extent to be resented by them (Power and Franck 2008: 637). This situation might indicate that, under the guise of FCC, institutional interests have taken precedence over what is in the interests of children, young people and families themselves and that health care practices may not be supportive of their needs. Parents of children with complex needs often perform a number of roles in caring for their child – being a parent and providing skilled 'nursing' care in addition to organising services and advocating for their child. There is, in fact an expectation that parents will undertake the role of health care provider, taking on care giving tasks outside of the 'normal' parenting role that were previously only undertaken within the domain of hospitals or other health care settings (McCann et al. 2012: 20). Many families experience significant care and financial burdens, including out of pocket expenses, care coordination and income loss (Kuo et al. 2012).

According to Shields (2010), FCC should not be about parents feeling pressured into undertaking all or part of the care for their child if they do not wish to, or if they are not able to. Parents should not be made to feel guilty when they do not undertake all or part of their child's care, whether this is out of choice or ability. FCC *is* about effective communication and negotiation with parents about their level of involvement and participation in their child's care: about what parents want to do and how capable they feel about undertaking aspects of care; about how often and how long they will be present; and the level of involvement they choose for active participation in decision making about their child's care (Shields 2010).

Family-centred care: where to for nursing children and young people?

Any suggestion that FCC should be abandoned as a way of working with children, young people and their families presents both moral and ethical challenges. Clearly barriers exist to implementing FCC in its fullest sense, yet surely it is something we should strive to achieve in our everyday practice as well as in the policies and guidelines that inform practice.

While caring relationships may be problematic, little is known about the meanings FCC holds for children's nurses. FCC as a philosophy of care originated in what Schön (1983: 42) described as the high, hard ground of research-based theory and technique. Application of the theoretical constructs of FCC in the 'swampy lowland' of practice has been shown to be problematic. What is required then if, in its ideal form, FCC is unachievable and cannot be implemented (Carter 2008)? Scholarly literature has a tendency to be dominated by the depersonalised, authoritarian voice and a negative or 'deficit view' of practice (Benner and Wrubel 1989: 395) that serves to limit and close discussion. One way that this distortion can be limited and congruence brought to the rhetoric of the literature around FCC and the realities of practice is through open dialogue. The challenge for children's nurses is to critically reflect on their practices and to engage in dialogue about their values, what underpins their care and how that is realised in practice.

A Practice Development Exercise by nurses on a paediatric unit in Australia has involved the nurses coming together to develop their values and what that means for their way of working together and with children, young people and families in child- and family- centred ways. The unit values include respect, communication, safety, partnership, teamwork and excellence (see Figure 1.4). The values are posted in a central area of the ward for all to see. More than this, however, there is discussion about the values in the nurses' everyday work, and the experiences of children, young people and families as compared to the values are actively explored. Children, young people and families have been surveyed and questions in the survey directly linked to the unit values. Findings from the survey have allowed the nurses to reflect on aspects of care that are positive and where experiences of children, young people and their families are congruent with the espoused values for family- and child-centred care. Nurses have also reflected on experiences that are less positive and where they may improve practices in order to improve the experiences of children, young people and families. Children's and parents responses to a survey provided important feedback to the staff about the views of those they care for in relation to the unit's espoused values of working with children, young people and their families in child- and family-centred ways. Areas highlighted in the work included communication and information, inclusion in care, opportunities for rest, activities and the physical environment. The work provided staff with an increased awareness of the needs of the children, young people and families, placing their interests at the centre of practice, and translated into a number of changes in response to their experiences, summed up in a quote from one nurse:

> I feel it helped us to really focus on the practical and simple changes we can make in our work to make this unit a better place for us, our patients and their families.

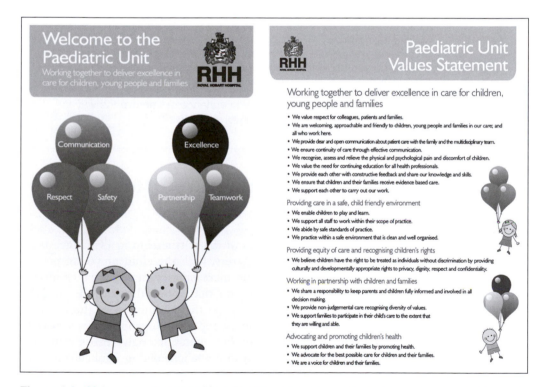

Figure 1.4   Unit values developed in a Practice Development Exercise considering family- and child-centred practice

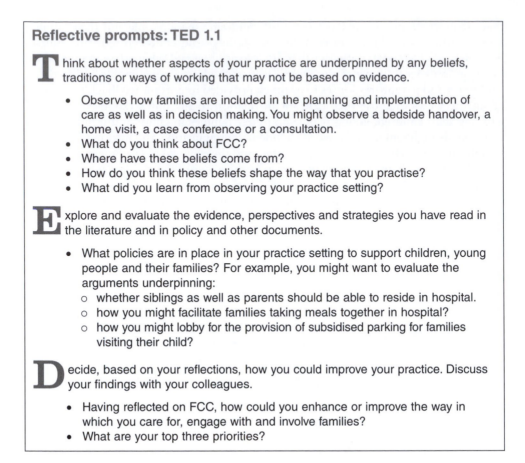

Reflective prompts: TED 1.1

Think about whether aspects of your practice are underpinned by any beliefs, traditions or ways of working that may not be based on evidence.

- Observe how families are included in the planning and implementation of care as well as in decision making. You might observe a bedside handover, a home visit, a case conference or a consultation.
- What do you think about FCC?
- Where have these beliefs come from?
- How do you think these beliefs shape the way that you practise?
- What did you learn from observing your practice setting?

Explore and evaluate the evidence, perspectives and strategies you have read in the literature and in policy and other documents.

- What policies are in place in your practice setting to support children, young people and their families? For example, you might want to evaluate the arguments underpinning:
  o whether siblings as well as parents should be able to reside in hospital.
  o how you might facilitate families taking meals together in hospital?
  o how you might lobby for the provision of subsidised parking for families visiting their child?

Decide, based on your reflections, how you could improve your practice. Discuss your findings with your colleagues.

- Having reflected on FCC, how could you enhance or improve the way in which you care for, engage with and involve families?
- What are your top three priorities?

Child-centred care: a further evolution in children's health care

Traditionally, the recognised active members of the partnership in FCC have been the health professional and the parents or carers, with the child or young person being allocated a more passive role. Yet the increasing recognition of children's active agency and right to participate has meant that we need to include children and young people as equals in the partnership, so that the notion of the child 'in family' rather than the child 'and family' may be the most appropriate way of conceptualising the relationship. This notion also resonates strongly with family systems nursing that focuses on the whole family unit when providing care (Wright and Leahey 1990). According to Wright and Leahey, who are credited with the presentation of the theory of family systems nursing, the '[c]oncentration is on both the individual and the family simultaneously... It is not "either/or" but rather "both/and"' (Wright and Leahey 1990: 149).

Child-centred care (CCC) means that children and their interests need to be at the centre of our thinking and our practice (Carter and Ford 2013). CCC also refers to the inclusion of children and young people as active participants in their care. CCC can be considered a further development in the on-going evolution of FCC or as an extension of the concept of FCC. According to Franck and Callery (2004: 269) the difference between FCC and CCC is one of emphasis and reflects the extent to which children's concerns are evidenced in the organisation of care. However, neither approach can exclude the other because CCC must take into account the social context in which children live, and FCC must have the health of children as a central concern. CCC acknowledges children as social actors in their own right. An important underpinning premise of CCC is the recognition that children's views are not always the same as those of their parents or of their health carers and that, when given the appropriate opportunities, children are able to represent themselves. FCC can mean that the child's voice is subsumed within that of their family's because professionals may assume that there is a shared family interest. However, this can present difficulties where this is not the case, such as when the child has a different viewpoint to the parents or in cases of child neglect or child abuse.

In contrast to traditional definitions of FCC, in CCC the child or young person is clearly positioned as a key and active member of the partnership. Underpinning this approach is the premise that the best interests of the child or young person must be the paramount consideration. Further, in a child-centred approach, health care professionals recognise children and young people as individuals with their own needs and rights to privacy and dignity, involving them in decisions affecting their care (Southall et al. 2000). Importantly, CCC still recognises the central role of parents and families in relationships and interactions with health care professionals, as evidenced in the examples for ways health services can be child centred (Figure 1.5). Work by Pritchard Kennedy (2012) shows how children in the study were clear that they wanted to develop their competence and become partners in care and in decision making.

As previously mentioned, it is also important to recognise the diversity and individuality of different childhoods and that children and young people are not an homogenous group. There is not one voice that speaks for children and young

---

- Consider the 'whole child', not simply the illness or condition
- Treat children as children, and young people as young people
- Be concerned with the overall experience of the child and family
- Treat children, young people and parents as partners in care
- Integrate and co-ordinate services around the child's and family's particular needs
- Graduate smoothly into adult services at the right time
- Work in partnership with children, young people and parents to plan and shape services and to develop the workforce

Figure 1.5   Principles underpinning child-centred health services (Department of Health 2003: 9)

people, nor is there one authentic account of children's lives, but rather there exists a diverse range of accounts (Christensen and James 2008). Children's lives, identities and experiences are shaped by many factors including age, gender, life experience, health, family background and friendship groups, school or nursery and their social, cultural, religious and economic situation (Carter and Ford 2013). In addition, children and young people face different opportunities and constraints and have different interests and preferences. For instance, in recognition of the specific cultural considerations of Maori Tamariki (children's) and Rangatahi (young people's) rights in health care, *The Charter on the Rights of Tamariki Children and Rangatahi Young People in Healthcare Services in Aotearoa New Zealand* (CHA and PSNZ 2010) recognises that while services are the same for every child and young person, specific actions are needed to address disparities in access to care.

Health care has been one of many contexts where children and young people have been denied rights of participation and their voices have gone unheard (Christensen and James 2008). Traditionally children and young people have been considered to lack expertise, experience, competence and capacity to be meaningfully engaged in their health care. Paternalistic attitudes where children are viewed as *becoming* (that is growing into adults), dependant, vulnerable and in need of protection can, in fact, result in their overprotection, disenfranchisement and exclusion. The meaningful and active involvement of children and young people in their health care through participation in choices and decision-making is something we are moving closer to achieving, rather than a space where we have truly arrived.

At the start of the values work described in Figure 1.4, it would not have been uncommon for the nurses just to survey parents' perspectives while not considering the perspectives of children and young people themselves. However, through reflection on their values the nurses on the unit enhanced their child-centred practice and now actively seek the voices of children and young people out of a concern to explore the children's experiences and the need to include them as well as parents as active and full partners in care. Children's and young people's responses reflect their own experiences of hospital; in the following examples issues of being bored and wanting choices are presented:

> This is my 3rd time in hospital in a couple of months in a way I would like more choices in meals or drinks. It would be good if rooms were sound proof. It can get boring really easily (13 years, 5 months)

> On the weekend I was bord but during the week I wasent as much and there were more ting to have fun with but they had to give me blood tests during the night (8 years)

Seeking the views of children and young people meant that their perspectives were heard, acknowledged and acted upon (where possible, given institutional or resource constraints). Their comments highlighted some areas of concern for them that were not necessarily noted by their parents, for example their comments regarding food choices and activities were not reflected in parents' responses.

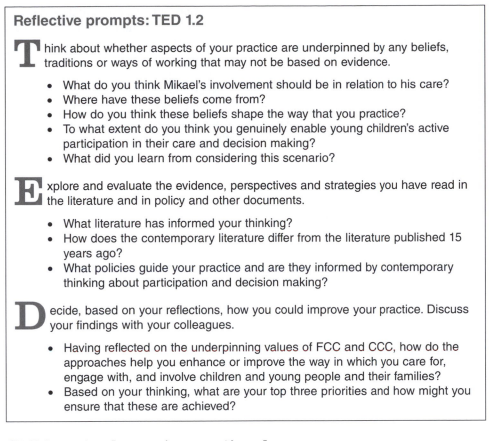

Reflective prompts: TED 1.2

Think about whether aspects of your practice are underpinned by any beliefs, traditions or ways of working that may not be based on evidence.

- What do you think Mikael's involvement should be in relation to his care?
- Where have these beliefs come from?
- How do you think these beliefs shape the way that you practice?
- To what extent do you think you genuinely enable young children's active participation in their care and decision making?
- What did you learn from considering this scenario?

Explore and evaluate the evidence, perspectives and strategies you have read in the literature and in policy and other documents.

- What literature has informed your thinking?
- How does the contemporary literature differ from the literature published 15 years ago?
- What policies guide your practice and are they informed by contemporary thinking about participation and decision making?

Decide, based on your reflections, how you could improve your practice. Discuss your findings with your colleagues.

- Having reflected on the underpinning values of FCC and CCC, how do the approaches help you enhance or improve the way in which you care for, engage with, and involve children and young people and their families?
- Based on your thinking, what are your top three priorities and how might you ensure that these are achieved?

Child-centred care in practice: how are we doing?

Although the standards cited in this chapter endorse children's and young people's participation in their health care as social actors in their own right, research indicates that children in many instances continue to have a marginal role in such processes (Coyne and Harder 2011: 313). Children's participation in decision making, choices and management of their care is the focus of Chapter 4.

Despite significant gains in children's hospital care since the last half of the 20th century, there is evidence of recent trends to reduce paediatric services. Even when separate facilities are provided, insufficient staffing and resources might mean that children are cared for alongside adults. For example, in Australia, where standards for the care of children and young people are in place, the co-locating of children alongside adults is common and often routine, despite evidence that this is not in the interests of child or adult (RACP 2009). Most paediatric emergency hospital presentations are to Emergency Departments in general hospitals, where children account for 20–30% of the total population of patients. A 2004 national survey of Australian health care settings found that some 35% of hospitals did not routinely accommodate children and young people separately from adults. Further, since 1992, the number of dedicated paediatric units had decreased by 30% (Hill et al. 2001: 81). Evidence would suggest that this situation has not changed since the survey was conducted. In Canada, only two of the 16 children's hospitals are now free standing following merges with adult or maternal facilities, a move that has been largely due to rising health care costs, rather than being specifically aimed at improving services for children (Stang and Joshi, 2006). These disturbing trends indicate not just a lack of progress towards child-centred health care services but, in some instances, a decline in such services.

Transitioning care: another consideration in the care of young people

As they mature children are expected to take on increasing self-care responsibilities and autonomy in relation to their health care. Being confident about self-care is of particular importance when young people with chronic conditions prepare for and move across to adult services. A strength of child-centred care, when it is working well, is that it can provide opportunities for young people to develop skills and competence to enable them to transition effectively. The best transition practices are underpinned by a collaborative, coordinated and integrative model that empowers young people and their carers. Structured transition programmes do occur but these are often confined to larger specialist settings. However, Doug et al. (2011) note the lack of an evidence base in most of the guidelines used to underpin the development of transition services. In work by Allen et al. (2012) a range of seven different 'continuities' – relational, longitudinal, management, informational, flexible, developmental and cultural – were identified as necessary to support smooth transition.

Improvements in technology and care mean that significant numbers of children with chronic conditions survive to adulthood, and transitioning from paediatric to mainstream adult services is an important milestone in the life of the young person. The transition from child/family-centred health care services to adult-oriented health services can present a challenge for young people and their families as well as for health professionals who provide care to them. This transition is not just an administrative event where a young person's patient file is handed over, but is in fact a complex undertaking that also needs to be a guided educational and therapeutic process (Department of Health WA 2009). Child-oriented and adult health systems are by their very nature quite different. Constraining factors that act as barriers to transition can include lack of infrastructure and precedence, lack of developmentally appropriate support and additional financial costs (Bennett et al. 2005: 373; RACP 2010). Paediatric services may 'hold onto' patients because of mistrust of adult services or because of a failure to promote a young person's independence and autonomy in health-care seeking. In addition, paediatric services are family-focused, while adult services treat patients as independent adults and are less engaged with the

wider family. This is problematic for young adults who still require family involvement because of the nature or severity of their condition or disability, or indeed
because this is their choice. Allen et al. (2011: 1000) talk of interdependencies
between young people and their parents and of 'how service structures are failing to
accommodate the fluidity of cross-generational relationships ... [and the need to]
develop service structures that recognize the continuing role played by mothers in
supporting their child with diabetes into early adulthood'.

As a result of the barriers that are in place in some settings, some young people
and their families may experience stressful and difficult transfers to adult care. These
arise when the transition is abrupt, unplanned or delayed so that they continue to be
cared for in paediatric services for longer than appropriate.

Conclusion

It is evident that the full participation and involvement of children, young people
and their families in the planning and delivery of their care requires careful attention
and on-going commitment by a wide range of people including health care professionals, policy makers and commissioners of services. Health care services need to
be designed around and responsive to the needs of children and young people, and
one way of moving closer to this is to see health care services through their eyes
(Department of Health 2003). The findings from the Bristol Inquiry are a clear and
sharp reminder of what can happen when children become the objects of care and
when the interests of children and families are not given primacy over institutional
and bureaucratic interests.

One of the aims of this chapter has been to challenge your thinking through the questions
and arguments presented, in order to encourage you to reflect on your nursing care of children and young people. Nurses caring for children and young people are in a position to
open up or close off opportunities for them and their families to be active participants in
their health care, including their participation in decision-making processes.

Acknowledgement

Thank you to Karen Demangone and Sue Lickiss, Diabetes Nurse Educators, Royal
Hobart Hospital for assistance in the development of the case study for this chapter.

References

Ahmann, E. (1994) 'Family centered-care: shifting orientation', *Pediatric Nursing*, 20(2):
113–117.
Allen, D., Channon, S., Lowes, L., Atwell, C. and Lane, C. (2011) 'Behind the scenes: the
changing roles of parents in the transition from child to adult diabetes service', *Diabetic
Medicine*, 28(8): 994–1000.

Allen, D., Cohen, D., Hood, K., Robling, M., Atwell, C., Lane, C., Lowes, L., Channon, S., Gillespie, D., Groves, S., Harvey, J. and Gregory, J. (2012) 'Continuity of care in the transition from child to adult diabetes services: a realistic evaluation study', *Journal of Health Services Research & Policy*, 17(3): 140–148.

Barnsteiner, J., Gillis-Donovan, J., Knox-Fischer, C. and McKlindon, D. (1994) 'Defining and implementing a standard for therapeutic relationships', *Journal of Holistic Nursing*, 12(1): 35–49.

Benner, P. and Wrubel, J. (1989) *The Primacy of Caring*. Menlo Park, CA: Addison-Wesley Publishing Company.

Bennett, D., Towns, S. and Steinbeck, K. (2005) 'Smoothing the transition to adult care', *Medical Journal of Australia*, 182(8): 373–374.

Carter, B. (2008) Commentary on Shields, Pratt and Hunter (2006) 'Family centred care: a review of qualitative studies', *Journal of Clinical Nursing*, 5: 1317–1323. *Journal of Clinical Nursing*, 17: 2091–2093.

Carter, B. and Ford, K. (2013) 'Researching children's health experiences: the place for participatory, child-centered, arts-based approaches', *Research in Nursing and Health*, 36(1): 95–107.

Carter, B., Cummings, J. and Cooper, L. (2007) 'An exploration of best practice in multi-agency working and the experiences of families of children with complex health needs. What works well and what needs to be done to improve practice for the future?', *Journal of Clinical Nursing*, 16(3): 527–539.

Children's Hospitals Australasia (2010) *Charter on the Rights of Children and Young People in Healthcare in Australia. Children's Hospitals*. Deakin: Children's Hospitals Australasia.

Children's Hospitals Australasia and Paediatric Society of New Zealand (2010) *Charter on the Rights of Tamariki Children and Rangatahi Young People in Healthcare Services in Aotearoa New Zealand*. Wellington: Children's Hospitals Australasia: Paediatric Society of New Zealand.

Christensen, P. and James, A. (2008) *Research with Children: Perspectives and Practices*, 2nd edn. London: Routledge.

Christensen, P. and Prout, A. (2005) 'Anthropological and sociological perspectives on the study of children', in S.M. Greene and D.M. Hogan (eds) *Researching Children's Experiences: Approaches and Methods*. London: Sage.

Coyne, I. and Cowley, S. (2007) 'Challenging the philosophy of partnership with parents: a grounded theory study', *International Journal of Nursing Studies*, 44(6): 893–904.

Coyne, I. and Harder, M. (2011) 'Children's participation in decision making: balancing protection with shared decision-making using a situational perspective', *Journal of Child Health Care*, 15(4): 312–319.

Darbyshire, P. (1994) *Living with a Sick Child in Hospital: The Experiences of Parents and Nurses*. London: Chapman and Hall.

Department of Health (2003) *Getting the Right Start: National Service Framework for Children and Young People: Standard for Hospital Services*. Central Manchester and Manchester Children's University Hospital NHS Trust.

Department of Health, Western Australia (2009) *Paediatric Chronic Diseases Transition Framework*. Perth: Health Networks Branch, Department of Health, Western Australia

Doug, M., Adi, Y., Williams, J., Paul, M., Kelly, D., Petchey, R. and Carter, Y.H. (2011) 'Transition to adult services for children and young people with palliative care needs: a systematic review', *Archives of Disease in Childhood*, 96(1): 78–84.

Ford, K. (2010) 'Reframing a sense of self: a constructivist grounded theory of children's admission to hospital for surgery'. Unpublished thesis, University of Tasmania.

Ford, K. (2011) '"I didn't really like it but it sounded exciting": admission to hospital for surgery from the perspective of children', *Journal of Child Health Care*, 15(4): 250–260.

Ford, K., Courtney-Pratt, H. and FitzGerald, M. (2012) 'Post-discharge experiences of children and their families following children's surgery', *Journal of Child Health Care*, 16(4): 320–330. &

Ford, K., Sankey, J. and Crisp, J. (2007) 'Development of children's assent documents using a child-centred approach', *Journal of Child Health Care*, 11(1): 19–28.

Franck, L.S. and Callery, P. (2004) 'Re-thinking family-centred care across the continuum of children's healthcare', *Child: Care, Health & Development*, 30 (3): 265–277.

Garling, P. (2008) *Final Report of the Commission of Inquiry: Acute Care Services in NSW Public Hospitals*. Vol 1. Sydney.

Hill, M., Pawsey, M., Cutler, A., Holt, J. and Goldfield, S. (2011) 'Consensus standards for the care of children and adolescents in Australian health services', *Medical Journal of Australia*, 194(2): 78–82.

Kennedy, I. (2001) *The Report of the Public Inquiry into Children's Heart Surgery at the Bristol Royal Infirmary 1984–1995: Learning from Bristol*. London: The Stationery Office.

Kuo, D., Houtrow, A., Arango, P., Kuhlthau, K., Simmons, J. and Neff, J. (2012) 'Family-centered care: current applications and future directions in pediatric health care', *Journal of Maternal and Child Health*, 16(2): 297–305.

MacDonald, M., Liben, S., Carnevale, F. and Cohen, S.R. (2012) 'An office or a bedroom? Challenges for family-centered care in the pediatric intensive care unit', *Journal of Child Health Care*, 16(3): 237–49.

McCann, D., Bull, R. and Wizenberg, T. (2012) 'The daily patterns of time use for parents of children with complex needs: a systematic review', *Journal of Child Health Care*, 16(1): 26–52.

Mikkelsen, G. and Frederiksen, K. (2011) 'Family-centred care of children in hospital – a concept analysis', *Journal of Advanced Nursing*, 67(5): 1152–1162.

Ministry of Health (1959) *The Welfare of Children in Hospital (The Platt Report)*. Central Health Services Council. London: HMSO.

Nicholson, S. and Clarke, A. (2007) *Child Friendly Healthcare – A Manual for Health Workers*. Nottingham: Child Friendly Healthcare Initiative. Available at: http://www.cfhiuk.org/publications/cfhi_manual.htm (accessed 14 April 2013).

Power, N. and Franck, L. (2008) 'Parent participation in the care of hospitalized children: a systematic review', *Journal of Advanced Nursing*, 62(6): 622–641.

Pritchard Kennedy, A. (2012) 'Systematic ethnography of school-age children with bleeding disorders and other chronic illnesses: exploring children's perceptions of partnership roles in family-centred care of their chronic illness', *Child: Care, Health & Development*, 38(6): 863–869.

Roets, L., Rowe-Rowe, N. and Nel, R. (2012) 'Family-centred care in the paediatric intensive care unit', *Journal of Nursing Management*, 20(5): 624–630.

Royal Australasian College of Physicians (RACP) (2008) *National Standards for Children and Adolescents in Health Care*. Sydney: RACP.

Royal Australasian College of Physicians (RACP) (2009) *Policy on the Co-Location of Adults with Children and Adolescents in Health Care Settings*. Sydney: RACP

Royal Australasian College of Physician (RACP) (n.d) *Transition to Adult Care Services for Adolescents with Chronic Conditions*. Sydney: RACP. Available at: http://www.racp.edu.au/page/paed-policy#adol&young (accessed 25 September 2013).

Schön D (1983) *The Reflective Practitioner*. New York: Basic Books.

Social Care Institute for Excellence (2008) '"Necessary stuff": the social care needs of children with complex care needs and their families'. Available at: http://www.scie.org.uk/publications/knowledgereviews/kr18-summary.pdf (accessed 2 April 2012).

Shields, L. (2010) 'Questioning family centred care', *Journal of Clinical Nursing*, 19(17–18): 2629–2638.

Shields, L., Pratt, J. and Hunter, J. (2006) 'Family centred care: a review of qualitative studies', *Journal of Clinical Nursing*, 15(10): 1317–1323.

Shields, L., Pratt, J., Davis, L. and Hunter, J. (2008) 'Family centred care for children in hospital (review)', *The Cochrane Collaboration*, Issue 3. Available at: http://www.thecochrane library.com/

Southall, D., Burr, S., Smith, R., Bull, D., Radford, A., Williams, A. and Nicholson, S. (2000) 'The Child-Friendly Healthcare Initiative (CFHI): healthcare provision in accordance with the UN Convention on the Rights of the Child', *Pediatrics*, 106(5): 1054–1064.

Stang, A. and Joshi, A. (2006) 'The evolution of freestanding children's hospitals in Canada', *Paediatrics and Child Health*, 11(8): 501–506.

Street, A. (1992) *Cultural Practices in Nursing*. Geelong: Deakin University.

United Nations (UN) (1989) *Convention on the Rights of the Child*, United Nations General Assembly, New York.

Wood, J. (2008) 'Bowlby's children: the forgotten revolution in Australian children's nursing', *Contemporary Nurse*, 30(2): 119–132.

Woodgate, R., Edwards, M. and Ripat, J. (2012) 'How families of children with complex needs participate in everyday life', *Social Science & Medicine*, 75(10): 1912–1920.

Wright, L.M. and Leahey, M. (1990) 'Trends in the nursing of families', *Journal of Advanced Nursing*, 15: 148–154.

Chapter 2

Children's and Young People's Position and Participation in Society, Health Care and Research

Key points

- Attitudes and practices towards children and young people in health care reflect the way they are positioned in society.
- Children and young people have traditionally been denied the rights to participate in their health care and their voices have gone unheard.
- Children's and young people's experience, status, rights and well-being are central to health care services to ensure their needs are met.
- Children's and young people's meaningful participation in research helps us develop more complex understandings of their experiences and can lead to improvements in care provision.

Key theories and concepts explored in this chapter include the changing nature of childhood, children's and young people's participation in care and research, and ethical implications.

Case study 2.1: Danny

Setting the scene

Danny is 15 years old and lives at home with his parents. He was diagnosed with Hodgkin's Lymphoma Stage 1 soon after his 15th birthday.

Danny was expected to have an excellent prognosis on completion of three cycles of chemotherapy. Each cycle entailed a three-week block involving one day of vincristine, doxorubicin and cyclophosphamide followed one week later by a second dose of vincristine. After a one-week break he was scheduled to return for another cycle and this was to be repeated three times therefore completing his course after nine weeks. Danny did not require any central venous access.

It was planned that Danny would have a PET scan (Positive Emission Tomography – a medical imaging scan) after completing three cycles and he would not require any further treatment thereafter.

(Continued)

(Continued)

Potential complications of his chemotherapy included alopecia, mild bone marrow suppression, cystitis, photosensitivity and nausea. However, minimal complications were anticipated in the recommended dosing.

Danny received his first cycle of chemotherapy as an inpatient in the children's ward. On the day he was due to start his second cycle he refused to leave home to go to the hospital or to have any further chemotherapy. His parents felt helpless and upset about the situation.

The Oncology Clinical Nurse Specialist met with Danny in the clinic setting and talked to him about the reasons he refused to go to the inpatient ward at the hospital for treatment. Danny was unhappy about chemo and the way it made him feel; his rapid hair loss and changes to his appearance; and having to go to the children's ward for chemotherapy. As a child Danny had a series of admissions to the children's ward in the hospital for treatment of severe eczema that included wet dressings, and this experience had a lasting negative effect on him.

The paediatric oncology team discussed possible alternative strategies in relation to Danny's care. This involved offering Danny the opportunity to have chemotherapy in the clinic setting, which would be facilitated by two nurses in the clinic adjusting their working hours.

The plan was accepted by Danny and he agreed to have the chemotherapy in the clinic. He was the only patient in the oncology clinic during his chemotherapy days, which had been organised to avoid the regular clinic treatment day. Danny was able to watch TV, use the hospital computer and sleep on the treatment room trolley.

Danny persevered despite a lot of nausea, which was both chemotherapy and anxiety induced and completed the three cycles of chemotherapy.

Danny later stated he much 'preferred having his chemotherapy in clinic and not in the hospital'.

That winter Danny returned to playing Australian Football League which he had not managed to do the previous season.

Introduction

The way that children and young people are currently positioned in society and health care reflects and has its origins in the changing ideologies of childhood and their status in the wider social world. The United Nations Convention on the Rights of the Child (UN 1989) and the acknowledgement of children and young people as active social beings and rights holders (Tisdall 2012) means we are now obliged to enable them to express their views on matters of importance to them. While the last two decades have seen the increased participation of children and young people in areas such as education, family law and in the development of public policy, it is only more recently that there has been an increased focus on their right to be heard in the context of health care (Donnelly and Kilkelly 2011). This change in focus compels health care professionals to find effective ways of engaging with children and young people that include listening skills, consultation practices and the inclusion of children and young people as active participants.

It is fundamental that children's nurses understand the lives of the children and young people they care for in order to provide nursing care that meets their needs. For health care services to be truly child-centred and to authentically respond to the needs of children and young people, their views and perspectives are crucial (Glasper and Evans 2013). Without effective engagement, adults are not able to access their perspectives, appreciate their concerns or meet their needs (Kellett 2011). Children and young people have critical and unique perspectives on their health and health care experiences, yet the inclusion of their perspectives on their care, policy and service development, and research about their perspectives of care has often been absent (Lansdown 2011). Adult views have traditionally informed policy and practice and the voices of children and young people have often been drowned out by those of adults speaking for and about them. Children's lives have typically been explored through the views and understandings of adult proxies including parents, professionals, policy makers, academics and researchers. There has been little acknowledgement that children's and young people's perspectives are 'separate to and different from those of their adult carers' (Cook and Hess 2007: 30). Children and young people have thus been rendered as 'objects' rather than active participants and they have been excluded from their health care planning and decision making as well as the research process (Christensen and James 2008). Child-centred care (CCC) and child-centred research reflects contemporary thinking and values that recognise children as social actors in their own right.

In this book, we refer to 'children and young people' as a broad and diverse group while acknowledging that childhood is characterised by different degrees of competence and a series of complex transitions (Hendrick 2008). So, rather than collectivising 'children and young people' and risk presenting a homogenised view of children and childhood, throughout the work we emphasise that each child and young person needs to be considered as an individual with particular perspectives, experiences and life-worlds.

In this chapter you will be able to reflect on your perceptions of children's and young people's agency and how children and young people are situated in health care and in research. You will also have an opportunity to think about how you might undertake practical activities in listening to children and young people and reflect on the impacts incorporating their views might have for practice.

Children and young people: their positioning in society and health care

> Childhood has its own way of seeing, thinking and feeling, and nothing is more foolish than to try and substitute ours for theirs. (Rousseau in *Emile*, 1792)

If Danny had been living in an earlier period of history, many aspects of his experience of illness and health care such as likelihood of survival, access to treatment, approaches to care, attitudes of health professionals and where his care took place would have been significantly different. Different orientations to childhood have existed over time and the following brief account of the positioning of children in different historical periods provides some perspective to the discussion on children's and young people's participation in health care and in research.

An historical perspective

In the Middle Ages there was little to distinguish children from adults and generally only two stages of development – infancy and adulthood – were recognised. Once over the age of 7 years, an individual was considered old enough to be physically independent of their parents. The more modern concept of 'childhood' emerged in the 18th century, influenced by the work of the 17th- and 18th-century authors Locke and Rousseau. Their works portrayed children as individuals in their own right, as can be evidenced by the quote from Rousseau above, but their works also influenced the views that children were unformed or 'becoming' persons, passive and dependent (Hogan 2005).

During the 19th century, Western society became increasingly aware of its responsibilities for the welfare of children, perhaps because of, or in light of, the appalling treatment of many children. Children came to be viewed as a special and vulnerable class in need of protection. Legislation was passed in Great Britain that aimed to protect children. This included: the Chimney Sweeps Act of 1840, banning the use of children as chimney sweeps; the Mines Act of 1842 forbidding the employment of women, girls and boys younger than 10 years underground; and the Education Act of 1870 which legislated for the universal education of children (Lansdown 1996). In segregating children from the adult world of work, schools became central to the construction of a new image of childhood.

In the first half of the 20th century, advice on raising children was influenced by the science of behaviourism – the belief that desired behaviours can be achieved by training children with rewards and punishments (Greig et al. 2007). In effect this meant that the parent and child were encouraged to be both physically and emotionally distanced from each other. American psychologist J.B. Watson (1928) provided typical parenting advice:

> There is a sensible way of treating children. Treat them as though they were young adults. Let your behaviour always be objective and kindly firm. Never hug or kiss them, never let them sit on your lap. If you must, kiss them once on the forehead when you say goodnight. Shake hands with them in the morning. Give them a pat on the head if they make an extraordinary good job of a difficult task. Try it out. In a week's time you will find how easy it is to be perfectly objective with your child and at the same time kindly. (Cited in Hughes 1999: 15)

However, significant shifts occurred in the 20th century in political, educational and social opinions regarding children's welfare and health. These changing views of children and childhood were influenced by developments including the emancipation of women, shifts in the economic infrastructure of family life and by the changing focus on research on children (Cunningham 2005).

The United Nations Convention on the Rights of the Child was adopted by the United Nations General Assembly in 1989 and it protects children's rights by setting standards in health care, education and legal, civil and social services (UN 1989). The Convention has had a wide-ranging and powerful impact on global views on children's status and rights, compelling adults to develop effective ways of including children as active participants in matters of concern to them.

Reflecting on the UN Convention, the development of children's rights and children's position in society in the 20th century, Carol Bellamy, Executive Director of the United Nations Children's Fund (UNICEF) stated: 'A century that began with children having virtually no rights is ending with children having the most powerful legal instrument that not only recognizes but protects their human rights' (UNICEF 2002). Although the UN Convention and other policies and charters outline the rights of children and young people, the actual protection of their rights needs to be made a reality. The vast majority of the world's children do not have their rights realised and so children continue to be harmed and remain unprotected.

The present

Societal and economic impacts provide varying contexts for children's lives in the 21st century. For example, in Western cultures, increasing numbers of children live in lone parent families and the higher proportion of older people presents issues for families and for society (Christensen and Prout 2005: 51). In Australia, the proportion of the population under 15 years of age in 2010 was approximately 20% and is estimated to decrease to be closer to 15% in 2050 (Commonwealth of Australia 2010: 10). Reasons for these changes include lower birth rates and increased life expectancy. Lower birth rates reflect increased choices available to women, access to education and employment, and higher living standards. Similar demographic changes are evident across other countries, including, for example, Japan (Ministry of Internal Affairs and Communications 2010) and Canada (Stang and Joshi 2006: 503). Population changes have implications for many spheres including health, labour force participation, housing and demand for skilled labour (Commonwealth of Australia 2011).

Other recent social phenomena that impact on children include their exclusion from public spaces and changes in play, activity and diet (Christensen and Prout 2005: 53; Darbyshire et al. 2005: 418). Obesity and diabetes, emotional, behavioural and mental health issues are increasingly impacting on the health and well-being of children and young people. Many children in countries that are adequately resourced do not have the recommended portions of fruit and vegetables in their diet or participate in the recommended 60 minutes of physical activity (or play) each day. In affluent countries, children spend increasing amounts of time watching television, at the computer or engaged in scheduled and structured physical activities such as ballet or soccer. They are participating less in active, unstructured and unsupervised outdoor play in the local neighbourhood or park, and this is thought to be impacting on their physical, emotional, social and cognitive development and well-being. Where once children played outside until called for dinner, this is less often the case due to concerns for safety or because of the structured activities they participate in after school. Children and young people also experience the impact of digital technology in their daily lives – they are often more proficient than adults in the use of mobile phones and computers, and engage in social networking and even 'second lives' in virtual worlds.

The level of protection (or as some may argue – overprotection), of children in Western cultures contrasts starkly with the experiences of those children across the world (including children in so-called advanced societies) who experience malnutrition, abject poverty, detention, conflict, child labour and prostitution. Children who experience poverty, for example, face many problems, including poor nutrition, poor environmental conditions, limited access to health care, worse outcomes from disease, and are less likely to have optimal health (Malat et al. 2005).There is an increasing recognition that the early years of a child's life have a profound impact on their future health, development, learning and well-being and productivity (Commonwealth of Australia 2010). Ironically, perhaps, one of the major drivers in the investment in the early development of children is an economic one, as governments recognise the contribution to work children will make in the future as adults. We would argue that this investment is necessary in the recognition of children and young people as equal citizens with equal rights now rather than only in the future.

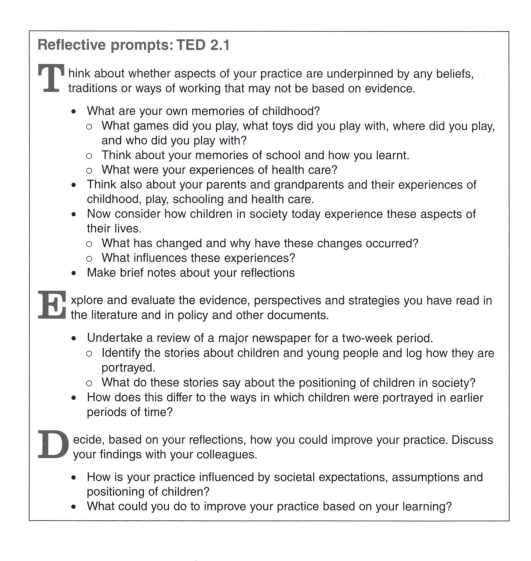

Reflective prompts: TED 2.1

Think about whether aspects of your practice are underpinned by any beliefs, traditions or ways of working that may not be based on evidence.

- What are your own memories of childhood?
  - What games did you play, what toys did you play with, where did you play, and who did you play with?
  - Think about your memories of school and how you learnt.
  - What were your experiences of health care?
- Think also about your parents and grandparents and their experiences of childhood, play, schooling and health care.
- Now consider how children in society today experience these aspects of their lives.
  - What has changed and why have these changes occurred?
  - What influences these experiences?
- Make brief notes about your reflections

Explore and evaluate the evidence, perspectives and strategies you have read in the literature and in policy and other documents.

- Undertake a review of a major newspaper for a two-week period.
  - Identify the stories about children and young people and log how they are portrayed.
  - What do these stories say about the positioning of children in society?
- How does this differ to the ways in which children were portrayed in earlier periods of time?

Decide, based on your reflections, how you could improve your practice. Discuss your findings with your colleagues.

- How is your practice influenced by societal expectations, assumptions and positioning of children?
- What could you do to improve your practice based on your learning?

Children's and young people's participation in health care

Just as children's and young people's positioning in society has changed over time, so too has their positioning in health care. Where they were once silent and passive recipients of care, children and young people are increasingly being heard and listened to as their perspectives are sought to inform policy and service delivery and as their active participation in their individual care is encouraged.

In the following quote from *The Strand Magazine*, we can only speculate on the views of the children who experienced surgery in the late 19th century.

> From the first ward we seek to enter we are admonished by our senses to turn back. We have barely looked in when the faint, sweet odour of chloroform hanging in the air, the hiss of the antiseptic spray machine, and the screens placed round a cot informs us that one of the surgeons is conducting an operation. The ward is all hushed in silence, for the children are quick to learn that when the big, kind-eyed doctor is putting a little comrade to sleep in order to do some clever thing to him to make him well, all must be quiet as mice. There is no more touching evidence of the trust and faith of childhood than the readiness with which these children surrender themselves without a pang or fear into the careful hands of the doctor. (From *The Strand Magazine*, 1891 cited in Lansdown 1996: 13)

The children's descriptions of their experiences are likely to be very different to the adult view presented here, yet we have no access to the children's perspectives, as they form no part of the historical record. The 'quiet as mice' children who 'surrender themselves without a pang or fear' in this silent ward were most likely extremely frightened of what might happen to them in a place where surgical procedures were performed behind the screens placed around their cots. From this description, it would also appear that parents had no presence in this hospital ward (Ford 2010).

A distinction can be made between 'hearing' what children say and 'listening' to what they say. Hearing is about the physical processing of sound, whereas listening is 'hearing with understanding' that also embodies respect and openness and incorporates an empowering construction that implies achieving change (Kellett 2011). There are also distinctions that can be made between consultation and participation. Children may be consulted with and yet what they have to say can still be ignored and they can be excluded from decision making. This kind of tokenism towards including children demonstrates a lack of respect for children and young people; neither fully acknowledging their rights nor recognising the important contributions they can make to improving practice and services. Participation is about doing and being involved, and their active participation requires children's and young people's meaningful involvement in decision-making processes (Kellett 2011). In addition to their right to participation in their health care, reasons for promoting children's and young people's views include providing a counterbalance to the dominant and prevalent voices of professionals and recognising that their views and experiences must be understood in order to provide services that meet their needs (Brotchie et al. 1998, cited in Caldwell 2004: 205).

There are instances where children and young people are harder to reach and are less able to voice their opinions and concerns and need to be given additional opportunities to be heard. Children and young people who are disenfranchised, vulnerable, or disengaged need to be supported and encouraged to participate in decision making. These disenfranchised groups include children and young people from indigenous populations, those with complex illness and disability, those with mental health problems, those in care, those with poor family support structures, the homeless and young offenders.

Children and young people with mental health problems present one group who require support to ensure they are empowered to the full extent to which they are able to participate in their treatment. Research shows that the incidence of mental health problems in Australian children is between 14% and 18%. Similarly, studies in countries such as New Zealand, Puerto Rico, United States and Canada indicate rates of 18% to 22% (Lennings 2003). Children's levels of participation can be influenced, for example, by whether the child or young person was instrumental or not in seeking treatment, or whether, because of their condition, they are actively engaged in their care and treatment or unaccepting of it (Macdonald et al. 2007).

Disabled children are also less likely to be involved in decision making, including decisions directly related to their health (Davey 2010). Disabled children are afforded limited opportunities to voice their views and health care professionals often find it difficult to effectively communicate with them; this can cause disabled children increased stress. As well as deep satisfaction and reward, nurses have expressed frustration and guilt when caring for children with special needs and the tensions they experience when unable to provide holistic care. Institutional pressures and pressures on time and resources mean that time for individualised care and attention is difficult to find (Ford and Turner 2001). A challenge for nurses and other health professionals when caring for a child who has complex needs, communication difficulties or severe learning difficulties, is to ensure that arrangements are made to establish their views (Hemsley et al. 2012). It should not be assumed that a disabled child is incapable of sharing in decision making. The issue is not whether a disabled child or young person can participate, but rather how they can do so.

Children whose first language is other than English also need to have consideration of their specific needs. Research in the US, Canada, the UK and Australia indicates that children whose first language is not English are less likely than those from an English speaking background (ESB) to access various forms of health care, including ambulatory, specialist and emergency care (Ou et al. 2010). These children and young people need to be enabled to be heard, and one way of achieving this is by providing access to appropriate interpreter services. Good access to such services will help ensure they and their parents are fully informed and understand information provided to them, and that they can effectively communicate their views, perspectives, choices and decisions to their health carers.

Tensions can arise when a child, the parents and professionals disagree on a treatment or plan of care, or when parents, in believing they are acting in the best interests of their child, request that information is kept from their child or that treatments proceed against the child's wishes. (This is considered in more detail in Chapter 3). It is also important to acknowledge that children need to be able to express their desire not to participate in certain choices or decisions; health professionals need to respect that position. In such circumstances, a leading premise in the decision-making process is what is in the best interests of the child. There is some critique of the concept of 'best interests of the child' as being vague, unknowable and potentially open to abuse (Hallstrom and Elander 2004: 368). The concept is, however, a fundamental principle of the UNCRC; it underpins the interpretations of all children's rights and needs to be a reference point to guide decisions about children's and young people's lives, including health care. Nurses who care for children and young people need to listen to *all* children and young people, and to advocate for their rights. How nurses respond to the views of children and young people and the 'impact, meaning and implications' (Caldwell 2004: 206) these views have for individual practice and services ultimately influences the experiences of care and care outcomes. The advocacy role includes protecting children's rights to self-determinism, enabling their participation in decision making and having their voices listened to (Hallstrom and Elander 2004).

Case study 2.2: Danny

Actively participating in decisions

Danny's case study is an example of how care practices can be responsive to children's and young people's needs. This can occur when children and young people are consulted on their experiences and perspectives of their health care, including their participation in clinical decision-making and their involvement as service-users.

Danny's previous experiences of health care clearly influenced his attitudes to, and concerns around, his current health care needs. Danny's experiences and fears were acknowledged and his preferences and choices were given precedence in care planning, while at the same time ensuring that he received the necessary medical treatment he required in a safe environment.

The clinical nurse specialist respected Danny's capacity to take part in the decisions and recognised him as an active partner, with his parents, in the team. This is in contrast to traditional relationships based on adults' power and control. Danny's right to be heard was realised in a very practical way that demonstrated respect for his preferences and choices and resulted in participation that was truly meaningful and authentic rather than tokenistic. In this practice example, Danny was placed at the centre of care. The way that the clinical nurse specialist engaged with Danny as an active participant, to ascertain his views and what he had to say, was a crucial part of the overall assessment, planning and delivery of his care. The nurse demonstrated sensitivity and skills to facilitate, support and promote his participation and this consultation process influenced the trust Danny felt and his eventual participation.

Careful care planning and changes to two nurses' work hours were required in order for Danny to receive his treatment in the outpatients unit. This scenario was also dependent upon an organisational culture of support that required resources and a preparedness to change the routine ways of working. Care for Danny involved his interests being at the centre of care, and his interests took precedence over institutional interests.

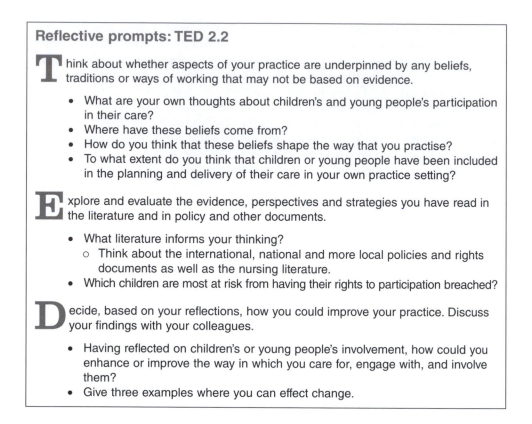

Reflective prompts: TED 2.2

Think about whether aspects of your practice are underpinned by any beliefs, traditions or ways of working that may not be based on evidence.

- What are your own thoughts about children's and young people's participation in their care?
- Where have these beliefs come from?
- How do you think that these beliefs shape the way that you practise?
- To what extent do you think that children or young people have been included in the planning and delivery of their care in your own practice setting?

Explore and evaluate the evidence, perspectives and strategies you have read in the literature and in policy and other documents.

- What literature informs your thinking?
  - o Think about the international, national and more local policies and rights documents as well as the nursing literature.
- Which children are most at risk from having their rights to participation breached?

Decide, based on your reflections, how you could improve your practice. Discuss your findings with your colleagues.

- Having reflected on children's or young people's involvement, how could you enhance or improve the way in which you care for, engage with, and involve them?
- Give three examples where you can effect change.

Children and young people's participation in research

Children's and young people's engagement in research is just one, albeit important component, in their participation in health care. However, since it is such a specific and important element, it is worth considering separately from their participation in their immediate health care. The impact that research *with* children and young people can have on the planning and provision of child-centred services forms a major feature of the discussion.

Until recently, little health research was genuinely child-oriented and research with children and young people was carried out on them, about them, or without them (O'Kane 2008: 126). Reasons for the absence of children's voices in research are many. Some of these reasons are similar to those relating to their lack of engagement in health care in general. Rather than engage with children, researchers approached parents/ carers and health professionals to gain insight into the life-worlds of children living with illness or disability (Irwin and Johnson 2005). Directly engaging with children was seen as unnecessary, too difficult and dangerous or likely to result in unreliable evidence as children were considered as lacking the required competence, experience and skills to be capable reporters of their lives (Campbell 2008; Lansdown 2011).

In addition, institutional ethical practices aiming to protect children from exploitation have tended to limit children's participation in health care (Skelton 2008). The summative result is that adults may have limited motivation to increase children's participation, yet without an authorial voice, children have little or no opportunity to contest adult accounts and children's voices remain 'muffled' (Hendrick 2008: 47).

The best people to provide information on the child's perspective, actions and attitudes are children themselves (Ford 2011; Mayall 2000). Children are needed to explain their world view, as argued by Christensen and James (2008: 9): 'Only through listening and hearing what children say and paying attention to the ways in which they communicate with us will progress be made towards conducting research with, rather than on, children'.

Children are increasingly recognised as being epistemologically privileged when it comes to research relating to matters of importance to children (Balen et al. 2006: 31). Adults, such as parents, teachers and health professionals, can provide important insights into children's behaviour. However, including children in research relevant to them provides a much more comprehensive account of the child's life (Scott 2008). In recent years, particularly within social science research, there has been a fundamental shift in understanding about children and a repositioning of them in research. Rather than being the objects of research, children are becoming more the subjects, or participants, and even researchers themselves. There is an increased understanding of children as 'social actors, communicators and meaning makers from the beginning of life, trying to make sense of their social world, in the various cultural contexts they inhabit' (Bruner and Haste 1987, cited in Woodhead and Faulkner 2008: 27). Such shifts have been less evident in health research.

Exploration of children's and young people's lives *without* their direct involvement means we fail to genuinely engage with and address children's own experiences of illness, disability or health care. It is increasingly recognised that adult perceptions of children's thinking, actions or needs can differ from what children themselves say. Where research has sought children's perspectives alongside those of adults (e.g., parents and health care practitioners) it is clear that children's views, opinions and perspectives are not always consistent with the adult view. This is demonstrated in a number of studies, including for example, work by Callery et al. (2003) on parents and young people's understandings of childhood asthma. Differences in perspectives and understandings were also identified by Madden et al. (2002) who explored children's and parents' (mother's) perspectives in relation to the children's experiences associated with renal disease. Relying on adult perspectives of children's experiences limits our ability to provide truly child-centred nursing practice and service delivery that is grounded in, and responds to children's needs. When children's accounts are presented, many taken-for-granted assumptions adults have about what children do think may be questioned.

There are various layers of participation and extents to which children and young people can be engaged. One of the earliest models to represent this was Hart's Ladder of Children's Participation (1992). The ladder has eight rungs – the first three represent forms of non-participation (manipulation, decoration and tokenism). The top five rungs represent varying degrees of children's participation (from being assigned tasks and being informed to sharing in decision making).

Another way of representing children's and young people's levels of participation is provided by Lansdown (2010) who identifies three levels of participation.

1. Consultative Participation – where children's views are sought to build under-standing of their worlds and experiences (an adult-led activity);
2. Collaborative Participation – where there is increased partnership between adults and children, with the opportunity for children's active involvement with aspects of a project (adults and children work in partnership);
3. Child-led Participation – where children initiate and lead an activity (as research-ers themselves with adults acting as facilitators) (Lansdown 2010: 20).

It may be appropriate to draw upon any one of these models of participation, depending on the nature of the study being undertaken. What is important is that the research involves the authentic engagement of children and young people, rather than a tokenistic approach to their involvement.

Ethical issues

Human research in general has contributed enormously to the human good and the vast majority of research is conducted in a safe and ethical manner (National Health and Medical Research Council (NHMRC) 2013). However, involving children in research can have unexpected consequences that do not always result in positive outcomes for children who are involved in that process (Naylor 2007). Research does have the potential to result in harm to children, and projects from the past serve as clear reminders of this.

In the 19th century, for instance, experiments on institutionalised children were common. In some instances children were deliberately infected with diseases includ-ing leprosy, syphilis and tuberculosis in order to study and test vaccines (Meaux and Bell 2001). In the Willowbrook Study in New York in the 1950s and 1960s, institu-tionalised children were injected with or ingested strains of hepatitis. This study involved coercion and deception as parents were given to understand their children were being vaccinated for hepatitis. There was also a waiting list for enrolment to the institutional school, and parents who consented to their child's participation in the study were immediately enrolled into the school (Johnson and Nelson 2000: 10). While most of the worst practices in relation to children being harmed in research are historical, it is only vigilance and care that ensures children currently in our care are not harmed by their involvement in research.

Ethical positions, like research approaches in general, have largely been designed for adults with untested relevance for research with children (O'Kane 2008). Ethical issues in research with children and young people relate in part to their understand-ings and experience of the world, which is different to that of adults, and also to the ways that children communicate.

Disparities in power relations between adults and children present a major challenge for conducting research with children that cannot be ignored in the research process. Indeed, structurally, children are made vulnerable because of a lack of political and economic power and civil rights as a result of historical attitudes and assumptions (Naylor 2007). The challenge for researchers working in contexts where children's voices have traditionally been marginalised, such as health care, is to find ways to overcome the power imbalance and to create spaces that enable children to speak out and to be heard (O'Kane 2008). Because adults have authority over them, children often find it hard to express dissent, to disagree or say things that they think an adult might find unacceptable. In addition, children are generally physically weaker than adults and usually have less well developed coping strategies. Many children are not used to being consulted or may feel their views are disregarded (Hill 2005). This perceived incompetence and weakness results in children being viewed as especially vulnerable to persuasion, influence and even harm – both in life and in research (Hill 2005). Carter (2009) critiques the default 'vulnerability' assigned to children in research that automatically frames and positions children, and can result in limiting their participation in research and knowledge of their perspectives. Ultimately adults have a continuing responsibility for ensuring the protection of children in research activities. Responsibilities include enabling children's participation in ways that are consistent with their interests, understandings and ways of communicating (Carter and Ford 2013).

Child-centred research approaches

As has been identified, children's participation in research is essential for theoretical, moral, ethical and practical reasons. Children are carriers of their own experience and research with children as participants is crucial if their needs are to be met. Acknowledgement of their diversity and individuality means that there are implications for the choice of research methodology and methods. Research that involves children as participants requires the use of special considerations, techniques and methods to ensure their interests are served. The child has different, although not inferior, abilities and competencies to adults and there are differences in power and abilities in terms of verbal competence and the expression and understanding of abstract ideas (Hill 2005). Just as children's understandings and experiences of the world are different to those of adults, so too are the ways that they communicate. The use of child-centred research methods can allow increased engagement with child participants (Carter and Ford 2013). Such methods incorporate the use of different and flexible methods of communication that are non-invasive and non-confrontational and can help to address ethical problems and power imbalances, and allow the child to inform, make decisions on, and also shape the research (Naylor 2007).

The health care environment is a context where children typically have little control. The creation of a safe, child-friendly physical space can facilitate children's and young people's participation and agency. Power differentials between children and adults include height, strength and language. Speaking to children from a standing position or from behind a desk accentuates the power imbalance. Sitting on a level with children is one way to help minimise this effect, either sitting on chairs or on the floor if appropriate. Physical strength can also be accentuated by body language and use of assertive gestures. Tone of voice and the use of accessible, cognitively appropriate language, the provision of explanations suited to the child's development and experience, and confirmation the child understands are other considerations in communicating effectively and respectfully.

Young children tire easily and have shorter attention spans, so frequent and shorter interactions are more appropriate than long interviews. Play-based activities that can be used with young children include story-telling, toys and puppets. Toys and puppets are valuable props that can provide safe vehicles through which to communicate with young children. Children in middle-school years may prefer group or individual interviews, and games-based methods. Young people may prefer focus groups (scheduled at a time to suit them), the use of graffiti boards, or engagement via mobile phone texts, chat rooms and blogs (Carter and Ford 2013; Kellett 2011). Arts-based methods have resonance with children's lives and day-to-day activities. Such methods can be effective ways to facilitate their engagement in discussion, control and interpretation of their experiences. Techniques include, for example, drawings and crafts or photographs taken by children and young people and provide ways other than the spoken word to communicate meaning. Arts-based techniques can help to broaden the different means of expression available to children and young people, and they can also help them to find the words needed to express themselves (Carter and Ford 2013).

Children as participants in research

Children's and young people's participation in research invites them to enter the dialogue, affords them recognition and respect and provides a way to explore the meanings, perceptions and understandings from their perspectives. Such research allows the views and experiences of children and young people to be considered in policy and practice, where planning and decisions concerning them are largely determined (Graham and Fitzgerald 2010).

The following examples present ways that the views of children and young people and their families can be sought in order to ascertain their experiences and needs so as to improve services and care provision. The examples illustrate just how change can come about on an international or national level or more locally in an individual practice setting.

There has been very little research about young people's own experiences of treatment – including the use of stimulant medication – for Attention Deficit Hyperactivity Disorder (ADHD). Although young people with ADHD are the primary consumers of the prescribed stimulant drugs, the necessity of these drugs is determined by adults. In recognition of the absence of young people's perspectives to date in this area, the National Institute for Clinical Excellence (NICE) guideline development group took the uncommon step of commissioning research with young people about their experiences of ADHD to inform the review of NICE Guidelines for ADHD (Singh et al. 2010). The researchers conducted a qualitative study using focus groups with young people with ADHD to explore their perceptions of, knowledge about, and attitudes towards stimulant medication. The research made an important contribution to the understandings of the role that methylphenidate can play in an individual child's family, educational and social life. The understandings were included in the reviewed guidelines and so have the potential to improve social outcomes, treatment adherence and therapeutic relationships between young people and their health care providers (Singh et al. 2010).

A study by Carter et al. (2012) is an example of how children with complex needs can be included as participants in research. The research focused on children's community nursing services for children with complex or special care needs and the researchers worked with children and young people and their families to identify what was working well in the service and how practices could be enhanced (Carter et al. 2012). The research included an advisory group with children and young people as members and workshops, interviews, blogging and emails to allow different ways in which the children and young people who were participating in the study could contribute their views. The research led to the incorporation of many of the findings into government legislation in England on Children's Community Nursing Services.

An example of the impact that research with children and young people can make to local care is a research project in a paediatric unit in Norway that aimed to implement a new education approach in the care for children with asthma. The qualitative study, using co-operative inquiry, included 90 participants (children, parents, health care professionals, teachers and students). Children were aged between 7 and 10 years, and using communication and research techniques adapted to the children's age, development and sensitivity, their perspectives were valued and taken into account during the period of intervention and influenced the changes made to asthma education practices in the unit (Trollvik et al. 2013).

Research demonstrates that children have varying experiences of being consulted and involved in their care (Coyne 2008), but the examples presented above show how powerful and sustainable change can be achieved by engaging with children and young people themselves at a more 'grassroots level' *in* practice. Nurses who work with children and young people need to be proactive in providing, facilitating and enabling children and young people to express their views. They also need to be innovative and sensitive to children's and young people's involvement and to be reflexive about how they engage children and young people.

Conclusion

Children are significant users of health care, their needs are different to those of adults, and their hospitalisation has physical, emotional and psychosocial impacts on them. In addition, political, social and economic contexts influence children's health care. There is a growing acknowledgement of children as persons in their own right who contribute to and shape their everyday lives and who are worthy of recognition, respect and voice. Further, children's experiences, status, rights and well-being are central to health care services for children.

In order for health care to more appropriately meet children's particular needs, understanding of children's perspectives is essential. This aspect of children's health care deserves attention, not only in light of international and national guidelines, policies and standards for children in health care, but also because of ethical and moral imperatives and children's fundamental rights. However, children's voices are not often listened to in either health care or research, and so there is a gap in our understanding of what the experience of health care means for children themselves.

Acknowledgement

Thank you to Helen Starosta, Clinical Nurse Consultant Oncology and Haemotology, Royal Hobart Hospital for her assistance in the development of the case study for this chapter.

References

Balen, R., Blyth, E., Calabretto, H., Fraser, C., Horrocks, C. and Manby, M. (2006) 'Involving children in health and social research: "human becomings" or "active beings"?', *Childhood*, 3(1): 29–48.

Caldwell, C. (2004) 'Practice development in child health nursing: a personal perspective', in B. McCormack, K. Manley and R. Garbett (eds) *Practice Development in Nursing*. Oxford: Blackwell Publishing, p. 200–21.

Callery, P., Milnes, L., Verduyn, C. and Couriel, J. (2003) 'Qualitative study of young people's and parents' beliefs about childhood asthma', *British Journal of General Practice*, 53(488): 185–190.

Campbell, A. (2008) 'For their own good: recruiting children for research', *Childhood*, 15(1): 30–49.

Carter, B. (2009) 'Tick box for a child? The ethical positioning of children as vulnerable, researchers as Barbarians and reviewers as overly cautious', *International Journal of Nursing Studies*, 46(6): 858–864.

Carter, B. and Ford, K. (2013) 'Researching children's experiences: the place for participatory, child-centered, arts-based approaches', *Research in Nursing and Health*, 36(1): 95–107.

Carter, B., Coad, J., Bray, L., Goodenough, T., Moore, A., Anderson, C., Clinchant, A. and Widdas, D. (2012) 'Home-based care for special healthcare needs: community children's nursing services', *Nursing Research*, 61(4): 260–268.

Carter, B., Marshall, M. and Sanders, C. (2009) 'An exquisite knowing of children', in R.C. Locsin and M. Purnell (eds) *Contemporary Process of Nursing: The (Un)bearable Weight of Knowing Persons in Nursing*. New York: Springer Publishing, pp. 281–303.

Christensen, P. and James, A. (eds) (2008) *Research with Children: Perspectives and Practices*. New York: Routledge.

Christensen, P. and Prout, A. (2005) 'Anthropological and sociological perspectives on the study of children', in S. Green and D. Hogan (eds) *Researching Children's Experience: Approaches and Methods*. London: Sage

Commonwealth of Australia (2010) *Australia to 2050: Future Challenges*. Attorney General's Department, Barton ACT.

Commonwealth of Australia (2011) Australian Demographic Statistics. June 2011. Available at: http://www.abs.gov.au/ausstats/abs@.nsf/0/AE3CAF747F4751CDCA2579CF000F9ABC (accessed 1 July 2013).

Cook, T. and Hess, E. (2007) 'What the camera sees and from whose perspective', *Childhood*, 14(1): 29–45.

Coyne, I. (2008) 'Children's participation in consultations and decision-making at health service level: a review of the literature', *International Journal of Nursing Studies*, 45(11): 1682–1689.

Cunningham, H. (2005) *Children and Childhood in Western Society since 1500*. Harlow: Pearson Education Limited.

Darbyshire, P. (1994) *Living with a Sick Child in Hospital: The Experiences of Parents and Nurses*. London: Chapman and Hall.

Darbyshire, P., MacDougall, C. and Schiller, W. (2005) 'Multiple methods in qualitative research with children: more insight or just more?', *Qualitative Research*, 5(4): 417–436.

Davey, C. (2010) *Children's Participation in Decision-making: A Summary Report on Progress made up to 2010*. London: National Children's Bureau.

Donnelly, M. and Kilkelly, U. (2011) 'Child-friendly healthcare: delivering on the right to be heard', *Medical Law Review*, 19(1): 27–54.

Ford, K. (2010) 'Reframing a sense of self: a constructivist grounded theory of children's admission to hospital for surgery'. Unpublished thesis, University of Tasmania.

Ford, K. (2011) '"I didn't really like it but it sounded exciting": admission to hospital for surgery from the perspective of children', *Journal of Child Health Care*, 15(4): 250–260.

Ford, K. and Turner D (2001) '"Stories seldom told": paediatric nurses' experiences of caring for hospitalised children with special need and their families', *Journal of Advanced Nursing*, 33(3): 228–295.

Franklin, A. and Sloper, P. (2005) 'Listening and responding? Children's participation in health care within England', *International Journal of Children's Rights*, 13(1–2): 11–29.

Glasper, A. and Evans, K. (2013) 'Supporting children and young people: the 15 steps challenge', *British Journal of Nursing*, 22(7): 422–423.

Graham, A. and Fitzgerald, R. (2010) 'Children's participation in research', *Journal of Sociology*, 46(2): 133–147.

Greig, A., Taylor, J. and MacKay, T. (2007) *Doing Research with Children*. Thousand Oaks, CA: Sage Publications.

Hallstrom, I. and Elander, G. (2004) 'Decision-making during hospitalisation: parents' and children's involvement', *Journal of Clinical Nursing*, 13(3): 367–375.

Hart, R. (1992) *Children's Participation from Tokenism to Citizenship*. Florence: UNICEF International Child Development Research Centre.

Hemsley, B., Balandin, S. and Worrall, L. (2012) 'Nursing the patient with complex communication needs: time as a barrier and a facilitator to successful communication in hospital', *Journal of Advanced Nursing*, 68(1): 116–126.

Hendrick, H. (2008) 'The child as a social actor in historical sources: Problems of identification and interpretation', in P. Christensen and A. James (eds) *Research with Children: Perspectives and Practices*. New York: Routledge, pp. 40–65.

Hill, M. (2005) 'Ethical considerations in researching children's experiences', in S. Greene and D. Hogan (eds) *Researching Children's Experiences: Approaches and Methods*. London: Sage Publications, pp. 61–86.

Hogan, D. (2005) 'Researching the child in developmental psychology', in S. Greene and D. Hogan (eds) *Researching Children's Experiences: Approaches and Methods*. London: Sage Publications, pp. 22–41.

Hughes, F. (1999) *Children, Play and Development*. Boston: Allyn and Bacon.

Irwin, L. and Johnson, L. (2005) 'Interviewing young children: explicating our practices and dilemmas', *Qualitative Health Research*, 15(6): 821–831.

Johnson, G. and Nelson, R.M. (2000) 'Informed consent and assent in human subject research', *Journal of Public Health Management and Practice*, 6(6): 9–18.

Kellett, M. (2011) 'Engaging with children and young people', *Centre for Children and Young People: Background Briefing Series*, no. 3. Lismore: Centre for Children and Young People, Southern Cross University.

Lansdown, G. (2011) *Every Child's Right to be Heard: A Resource Guide on the UN Committee on the Rights of the Child General Comment No 12*. London: Save the Children's Fund. Available at: http://www.unicef.org/adolescence/files/Every_Childs_Right_to_be_Heard.pdf (accessed 1 July 2013).

Lansdown, J. (1996) *Children in Hospital*. Oxford: Oxford University Press.

Lansdown, J. (2010) 'The realisation of children's participation rights', in B. Percy-Smith and N. Thomas (eds) *A Handbook of Children and Young People's Participation: Perspectives from Theory and Practice*. Abingdon: Routledge, pp. 11–23.

Lennings, C. (2003) 'Assessment of mental health issues with young offenders'. Paper presented at the Juvenile Justice: From Lessons of the Past to a Road for the Future Conference convened by the Australian Institute of Criminology in conjunction with the NSW Department of Juvenile Justice, Sydney, 1–2 December.

Liddell, K. and Hall, A. (2005) 'Beyond Bristol and Alder Hey: the future regulation of human tissue', *Medical Law Review*, 13(2): 170–223.

Macdonald, E., Lee, E., Geraghty, K., McCann, K., Mohay, H. and O'Brien, T. (2007) 'Towards a developmental framework of consumer and carer participation in child and adolescent mental health services', *Australasian Psychology*, 15(6): 504–508.

Madden, S., Hastings, R. and Hoff, W. (2002) 'Psychological adjustment in children with end stage renal disease: the impact of maternal stress and coping', *Child Care, Health & Development*, 28(4): 323–330.

Malat, J., Oh, H.J. and Hamilton, M. (2005) 'Poverty experience, race and child health', *Public Health Reports*, 120(4): 442–447.

Mayall, B. (2000) 'Conversations with children: working with generational issues', in P. Christensen and A. James (eds) *Research With Children: Perspectives and Practices*. London: Falmer Press, pp. 120–135.

Meaux, J.B. and Bell, P.L. (2001) 'Balancing recruitment and protection: children as research subjects', *Issues in Comprehensive Paediatric Nursing*, 24(4): 241–251.

Ministry of Internal Affairs and Communications (2010) The Statistics Bureau and the Director-General for Policy Planning of Japan: Population Census. Available at: http://www.stat.go.jp/english/data/kokusei/index.htm (accessed 16 February 2010).

National Health and Medical Research Council (NHMRC) (2013) *National Statement on Ethical Conduct in Human Research*. Australian Government.

Naylor, A. (2007) '"Every Child Matters": ethical and methodological considerations in studying children's early childhood experiences', *Educational Futures*, 16–41.

O'Kane, C. (2008) 'The development of participatory techniques: facilitating children's views about decisions which affect them', in P. Christensen and A. James (eds) *Research With Children: Perspectives and Practices*. New York: Routledge, pp. 125–155.

Ou, L., Chen, J. and Hillman, K. (2010) 'Health services utilisation disparities between English speaking and non-English speaking background Australian infants', *BMC Public Health*, 10: 182. Available at: www.biomedcentral.com/1471-2458/10/182 (accessed 1 April 2013).

Rousseau, J. (1762) "Emile" in *Education: Ends and Means* (1997, J. Sigler ed.). Lanham, MD: University Press of America, pp. 181–216.

Scott, J. (2008) 'Children as respondents: the challenge for quantitative methods', in P. Christensen and A. James (eds) *Research With Children: Perspectives and Practices*. New York: Routledge, pp. 87–108.

Singh, I., Kendall, T., Taylor, C., Mears, A., Hollis, C., Batty, M. and Keenan, S. (2010) 'Young people's experience of ADHD and stimulant medication: a qualitative study for the NICE Guideline', *Child and Adolescent Mental Health*, 15(4): 186–192.

Skelton, T. (2008) 'Research with children and young people: exploring the tensions between ethics, competence and participation', *Children's Geographies*, 6(1): 21–36.

Stang, A. and Joshi, A. (2006) 'The evolution of freestanding children's hospitals in Canada', *Paediatrics and Child Health*, 11(8): 501–506.

Tisdall, E.K (2012) 'The challenge and challenging of childhood studies? Learning from disability studies and research with disabled children', *Children & Society*, 26(3): 181–191.

Trollvik, A., Eriksson, B., Ringsberg, K. and Hummelvoll, J. (2013) 'Children's participation and experiential reflections using co-operative inquiry for developing a learning programme for children with asthma', *Action Research*, 1(1): 31–51.

United Nations (UN) (1989) *Convention on the Rights of the Child*. New York: United Nations General Assembly.

UNICEF (2002) United Nations Special Session on Children. Available at: http://www.unicef.org/specialsession/rights/path.htm (accessed 21 April 2013).

Woodhead, M. and Faulkner, D. (2008) 'Subjects, objects or participants? Dilemmas of psychological research with children', in P. Christensen and A. James (eds) *Research with Children: Perspectives and Practices*. New York: Routledge, pp. 10–40.

Chapter 3

Consulting and Informing Children and Young People

Key points

- This chapter will examine how information is discussed, shared and provided to children, young people and parents in relation to health care.
- Different methods of giving, receiving and sharing information will be discussed along with how different settings can influence the exchange of information.
- Information sharing underpins the education and preparation of children and young people and their parents for procedures, health care encounters and the management of long-term conditions.
- The information needs and priorities of children, young people, their parents and health professionals can differ.

Key theories and concepts explored in this chapter are methods of information sharing, engaging with children, young people and their families in health care settings and preparing children and young people for procedures, interventions and condition changes.

Case study 3.1: Jayden

Setting the scene

Jayden is 8 years old and has been admitted with acute tummy pain and vomiting for three days. He is dehydrated and in pain. His mum (Alison) and grandma are with him and Jayden is sitting on his mother's knee looking worried, tired and withdrawn. Despite being in pain and wincing when his tummy is pressed, Jayden lets the doctor examine him. The nurse undertakes and records his observations while he cuddles into his mother. It is suspected he has appendicitis and he needs to have bloods taken and an intravenous (IV) cannula inserted to administer pain relief and IV fluids as he is Nil By Mouth. Jayden has fallen asleep on Alison's knee and does not hear the doctor discussing the planned treatment. Alison is not keen to tell Jayden that the doctor needs to put in an IV cannula as he had a bad experience of immunisations within the General Practitioner (GP) setting. Alison describes Jayden as now being needle phobic. When Jayden wakes up he hears the nurse say they will do the IV in the next 20 minutes. In between periods of pain, Jayden states that he 'just wants to be better' and 'doesn't want to know what the doctors are going to do to him' but he is asking 'what is this cream on my hand and arm for?'

Introduction

This chapter will examine how information is discussed, shared and provided to children, young people and their parents in relation to health care. Different methods of information provision will be discussed and consideration will also be given to how different settings can influence the sharing of information. Information sharing underpins the education and preparation of children and young people and their parents for hospitalisation, management of long-term conditions and changes to health status. The different information and education needs within families will be discussed along with opportunities and challenges in communicating with children, young people and families.

Gaining and sharing information

The sharing and receiving of information is a fundamental part of everyday human life and is something that we do thousands of times a day, often without much thought. Information exchange through seeking, giving, verifying or clarifying information (Cegala et al. 1998) relies on communication through face-to-face interaction, written information or through supportive media such as the internet or telephone.

Information underpinning interactions

Children and young people are constantly engaged in information sharing in structured situations such as school classrooms and health provision, as well as in daily interactions with parents, family members, peers or through radio, television and the internet. However, children and young people who can communicate effectively in everyday life can often be excluded from effective information sharing within health care interactions due to the attitudes of adults to their inclusion and the dominance of medical terminology or language (Lambert et al. 2008; Tates and Meeuwesen 2001). Communication within health care is similar yet different from normal social interactions as the discussions can involve intimate, private and upsetting information (Levetown 2008), which children and young people may be excluded from or unprepared to discuss themselves. As effective communication underpins all diagnosis, treatment and care, poor health-related communication can result in compromised outcomes for patients and their families and prompt lifelong anger and regret (Levetown 2008).

Historically, the provision of information was directed primarily to parents during the very limited times that parents were allowed to visit the hospital and see their children. Although, in many cases, contact and communication between families and professionals has improved, the inadequate provision of information to children and parents continues to be highlighted as a key finding by national enquiries (Bristol

Royal Infirmary Inquiry 2001). Evidence from the United States of America has shown that from 35–70% of legal cases involving poor care within the health service relate to incidences where services and professionals have delivered poor levels of information and have failed to understand patient and family perspectives (Levetown 2008). In order for parents to fulfil their caring responsibilities they need 'the fullest account of what is proposed, the alternatives, the risks and possible outcomes' (Bristol Royal Infirmary Inquiry 2001; Chap. 29, para. 18).

There is an increasing recognition that children and their own young people are competent reporters on their own lives (James and Prout 2004) and their own health and, as such, their perspectives should be heard during health care interactions (Coyne and Kirwan 2012). The United Nations Convention on the Rights of the Child states that children have the right to have their views heard and respected (UN General Assembly 1989). The historical belief that children should be '*seen and not heard*' has hopefully passed, and children and young people are increasingly being encouraged to be involved in information sharing and consultations. As a result of the impact of acknowledging children's rights in this area, there is a lesser or different emphasis placed on professional and parental voices, and greater recognition of children's and young people's developing competencies and abilities to accurately recall and report on medical information. Involving children and young people with long-term conditions in information sharing and condition management enables them to gain knowledge and competence in dealing with their condition, something they will be increasingly expected to do as they develop into adolescence and adulthood (Stinson et al. 2008).

Providing information in an appropriate way to children, young people and their parents can be a complex process. In many cases information can be withheld or not discussed for fear of causing upset or anxiety to children. The withholding of information from children is not supported by evidence and children have demonstrated that even when a difficult diagnosis has purposefully been withheld from them, they were aware of their terminal illness diagnosis and prognosis (Bluebond-Langner 1978). Children and young people can quickly perceive in many cases when the truth or information is being withheld from them (Bray et al. 2012; Young et al. 2003) and by using whatever information they have (even when this is incomplete or inaccurate) children will continually try to make sense of their situation (Levetown 2008). Parents intuitively try and protect their children from any harm they may encounter and to reduce any upset; this relates to both day-to-day life and particular circumstances such as within health services. It seems that having sensitive honest conversations can be less upsetting and better promote trusting relationships than withholding information. Despite this, many parents continue to choose not to disclose information to their children and act as information executors, monitoring and concealing certain information. and, in these cases, providing information within a 'family-centred' model can be challenging.

Different family members may often have different needs for information, for example parents may wish to know a lot of information about the possible side effects of a prescribed medication, but not want to scare their child or put them off taking it. This may mean that parents go away from a consultation without discussing all the information they wanted or, alternatively, their child sits through the consultation listening to a list of off-putting possible side effects. In contrast parents may choose not to want to know 'the ins and outs' of a proposed treatment and as a result exclude their child from opportunities to receive this information. This 'mismatch' between individuals' health information seeking behaviours and the needs of other family members (Lambert and Loiselle 2007) can result in difficult, strained and sub-optimal consultations and engagement. The following example relates to a mother whose daughter was undergoing surgery for a long-term continence condition, who describes her approach to gaining information about the operation and an assumption that her daughter has similar beliefs:

> She doesn't like knowing, she is like me. You can take me in and do whatever you want to me, but just don't tell me about it first. So she is very much like 'all I want to know is how long I'm going to be in and when I'm going to be out and am I going to be alright when I'm done'. Then we said 'we don't want to know actually how they were going to do the operation, we don't want to know all the gory bits, just is it right for her and is it going to work for her. (Sarah's mother) (Bray 2010: 137)

Such attitudes can make it difficult for health professionals to ensure that children, young people and their parents know about proposed treatment and are fully

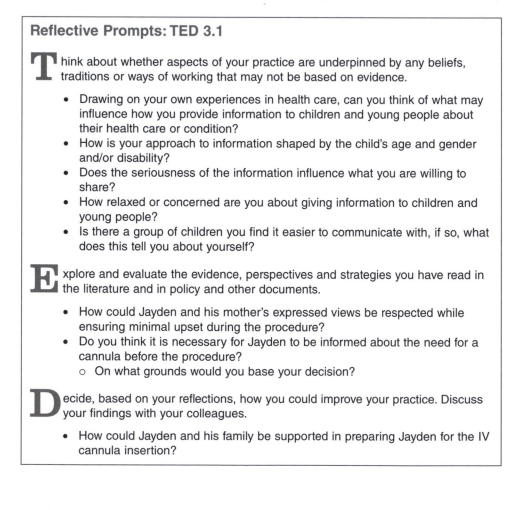

Reflective Prompts: TED 3.1

Think about whether aspects of your practice are underpinned by any beliefs, traditions or ways of working that may not be based on evidence.

- Drawing on your own experiences in health care, can you think of what may influence how you provide information to children and young people about their health care or condition?
- How is your approach to information shaped by the child's age and gender and/or disability?
- Does the seriousness of the information influence what you are willing to share?
- How relaxed or concerned are you about giving information to children and young people?
- Is there a group of children you find it easier to communicate with, if so, what does this tell you about yourself?

Explore and evaluate the evidence, perspectives and strategies you have read in the literature and in policy and other documents.

- How could Jayden and his mother's expressed views be respected while ensuring minimal upset during the procedure?
- Do you think it is necessary for Jayden to be informed about the need for a cannula before the procedure?
  - On what grounds would you base your decision?

Decide, based on your reflections, how you could improve your practice. Discuss your findings with your colleagues.

- How could Jayden and his family be supported in preparing Jayden for the IV cannula insertion?

prepared for interventions. This family encountered complications following surgery and became very upset, feeling that they had '*gone in blind*' to the procedure, even though this had been their expressed preference at the time.

Conversations and difficulty in sharing information within families can be particularly difficult when a terminal or life limiting illness has been diagnosed. One study identified that bereaved parents who chose not to speak to their terminally ill children about dying displayed regret and increased incidence of depression after their child's death than those who spoke openly with their children (Kreicbergs et al. 2004). It may be that parents prefer to hear information about life-threatening conditions without the child in the first instance so they can compose themselves and portray a strong parent identity for their child without breaking down or getting upset (Young et al. 2003).

Information about more than the condition

Health professionals are reported by parents as the main source of information about their child's condition, although health professionals may understand more about physiological processes than the psychosocial impact of health conditions. It can be difficult for professionals to know, or they may not be interested in knowing, about children's, young people's or families' everyday lives and the complex relationships, roles and aspirations within a family unit. However, this information is important in some cases to judge the true impact of health treatments (Bray et al. 2012) and how these can be incorporated into school, social and family life. Specifically, doctors have been criticised for focusing on the child's medical condition during interactions, with the child being of secondary importance (Beresford and Sloper 2003). It is suggested that to address this, children and young people with long-term conditions should have an annual meeting with the health care team to discuss the 'big picture' of their condition including social issues, school, peer and family support (Perrin et al. 2000). Within the UK, the Early Support Services Initiative aims to actively support how information is provided to families whose child has a disability, and this relates particularly to early and on-going information provision on conditions and local services (Department for Education and Skills and the Department of Health 2003).

The wider issues associated with condition management can be the main areas of concern for children coping with a long-term condition and their parents. Information relating to the emotional effects of a long-term condition, how to talk to friends about conditions and how to 'fit in' at school and with friends are of primary importance to young people with long-term conditions (Stinson et al. 2012). These are often conversations which do not take place within health care consultations. Time constraints and a focus on the physical aspects of condition management can leave children and their parents seeking information from other less reliable sources. Specifically, young people have identified that it is often the broader lifestyle questions and sensitive or personal information which can be the most difficult to ask health professionals (Beresford and Sloper 2003; Sanders et al. 2011) and which health professionals feel least equipped to deal with (Bray et al. 2012).

Different methods of gaining and sharing information

There are many different ways that children, young people and their parents gain and share information within the health service. Interactions often occur within planned consultations, but information is also shared in less structured settings including wards, emergency departments, homes and schools.

Consultations and sharing information from health professionals

Health professionals are often the key source of health information for parents, children and young people. Children with health conditions and their parents have identified that health professionals at general practitioner clinics (Khoo et al. 2008) or specialised health clinics are their most common source of support and information (Stinson et al. 2012), followed by internet websites and family and friends (D'Alessandro et al. 2004; Stinson et al. 2012). The most common setting for health-based communication and information sharing is in a planned consultation in an outpatient or primary care setting, although, as highlighted above, information is shared between parents, children and health professionals in many different contexts including home, school and inpatient and emergency settings in acute care.

Children and young people can be marginalised in consultations with their voice being lost to the more dominant adult voices (parents and health professionals) (Cahill and Papageorgiou 2007; Savage and Callery 2007; Tates and Meeuwesen 2001). Children have described boredom and a passive 'sitting through it' attitude to consultations about their health condition (Savage and Callery 2007), or they attempt to engage in medical consultations using language picked up from the adults; however, their efforts to report their subjective experiences of illness are often squashed by the adults present (Nova et al. 2005). Professionals in consultations can unintentionally position themselves in a way which children perceive as unapproachable and with little active engagement (Figure 3.1).

Even when health professionals attempt to engage with children and young people directly, parents can interrupt their child's response (Tates and Meeuwesen 2000), parents' responses may be privileged over their children's (Savage and Callery 2007), questioning and dialogue only relates to non-medical everyday chit chat (Aronsson and Rundstrom 1989; van Dulmen 1998), or children's accounts are questioned and not believed (Carter 2002). It is not enough just to hear children, but their views should be listened to and taken into consideration.

This marginalisation can represent the experiences of children and young people who have minimal contact with health professionals as well as those who have established long-term relationships (Beresford and Sloper 2003; Cahill and Papageorgiou 2007). Although interactions with children and young people within

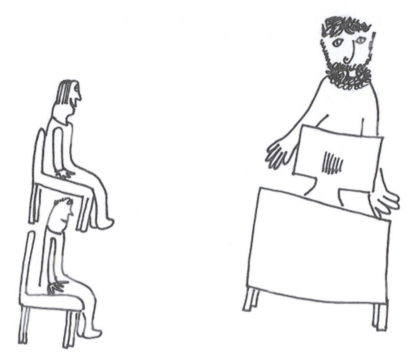

Figure 3.1   A 6-year-old's drawing of his appointment with a consultant

planned health care consultations are improving from the time when children were not expected to participate or even be present, there still remains a disparity in how they are afforded the opportunity to report on their lives (Tates and Meeuwesen 2001). It has been reported that children are involved in less than 10% of the total interaction, with even older children being minimally involved (Nova et al. 2005). Initiatives such as the 'toolkit for child centred asthma care' (Callery and Milnes 2012) have aimed to address the difficulties children and young people can experience in having their voice heard during consultations. This resource was evaluated as able to provide structure through a child diary and an interview schedule which focused health professionals' focused their information seeking and sharing directly on the children and young people. The focus remained on children and young people even when parents attempted to assert control through interrupting and overriding the information their children provided (Callery and Milnes 2012).

There is more known about communication and how information is shared within planned clinic consultations and less about how children, young people and their parents are communicated with in less formal environments, such as with health professionals during inpatient stays, in their homes, schools and in unplanned or emergency interactions in hospital. Suggestions of how to engage with children and young people within any health setting are presented in Table 3.1. There are accounts within the literature where parents have been provided with devastating news of their child's death by health professionals in corridors or other general clinical areas (Jurkovich et al. 2000) and it is hoped that these are rare instances and more appropriate approaches underpin practice.

Communication and information sharing can be complicated when those present do not have a shared language (Gibson et al. 2005). In these instances interpreters are relied on to relate information from parents to health professionals, which can cause children's and young peoples' voices to be further relegated to the periphery of consultations. The everyday practice of an English-speaking child member of the family acting as a translator is not appropriate in health care interactions where it is important for accurate and often complicated information to be relayed and also where the child themselves may be upset or emotionally influenced by the information being shared (Levetown 2008). Cultural considerations may influence how information is communicated and discussed with a family, and different cultures may have different practices regarding who is spoken to within the family (Levetown 2008).

Parents and children should ask as much about a treatment as possible, and one recommendation is that they use a notebook to write down any questions to make the most out of any health care consultations. The National Service Framework (DH 2004) in the UK advocates the use of audio recordings during consultations to improve communication and recall of the discussion, especially when complex and difficult information is being shared. Evidence suggests that recording conversations

Table 3.1   Strategies to engage with children and young people in the health setting (based on Levetown 2008)

- Speak with children and young people, not at or to them.
- Use accessible language to engage with children and young people.
- Speak in a quiet setting and seek to use child-friendly spaces.
- Ask children and young people who they would like to be present during consultations or interactions.
- Be interested in the child or young person as a whole and not just their condition or illness.
- Allow children and young people to have time to think through information and then time to ask questions.
- Engage with children by sitting next to them, not at a distance or height or from behind a desk.
- Listen actively to what they have to say.
- Pay attention to non-verbal expressions such as body language and facial expressions.
- Use drawings, games or other creative communication tools.
- Recognise that different agendas and needs may exist within a family.
- Ask the child what he or she would do with three wishes or a magic wand.
- Avoid potentially threatening gestures.
- Consider the welcome children and young people receive on entry to the service.

can aid the understanding of information provided to patients with cancer or their parents (Bruera et al. 1999; Eden et al. 1993), but it is unclear how widely this is used outside research studies. Health professionals can often rely on parents to ask the relevant questions to obtain the information they need (Bray et al. 2012; Gibson et al. 2005), but in many cases it can be difficult for parents to know what to ask when they have limited information about a condition or treatment options. Also it has been suggested that 'children should be told as much as they want to know' (Wollin et al. 2004: 131), but this in itself can be difficult to judge. Where a large quantity of complex information needs to be provided it may be more appropriate that this is not all squeezed into one consultation, but that families are given the opportunity to go away and process some information and discuss options between themselves before returning for a second consultation.

As well as face-to-face interaction between children, young people, their parents and health professionals, there are many others ways in which information is sought, provided and received.

Written and visual information

Written leaflets are a common way for information to be given to children, young people and particularly parents. These can take the form of hospital written leaflets (Lewis et al. 2012), narrative story books (Scott et al. 2012), manufacturers' leaflets relating to medication, or charity or company information about specific conditions or support mechanisms. Much of this information is focused on parents, but increasingly specific information is being written for children and young people (Felder-Puig et al. 2003; Trollvik et al. 2013). It is important to have distinct information as children and young people will use different words and expressions for conditions and treatment depending on their developmental level, and will need information presented in a different way from adults. The use of illustrations and pictures can help to make information more accessible and engaging and has been shown to help children and young people remember information more easily (McGuigan and Salmon 2005). Children, particularly younger children, may relate better to and feel more comfortable engaging with visual images as they may lack the written or spoken vocabulary to gain and share information from material reliant on written text.

Some written information for children with asthma has been designed by children during consultation exercises aiming to ensure that educational material is relevant and children and young people can relate to the content and that it is meaningful to them (Trollvik et al. 2013). This information uses stories and pictures to give condition-specific information but also to encourage children to learn problem-solving skills to equip them in managing their condition day to day in school, home and wider social situations. It is important to recognise that information designed for children may not be relevant to young people, and the use of pictures and material targeted specifically at children can cause young people to become disengaged and seek alternative, possibly less reliable, sources of information.

Although written information can be an important method of conveying information, it is important that information is supplied in a variety of formats, media and languages (DH 2004). The provision of a leaflet is seen as a simple and quick task and it is not always ascertained if the parent, child or young person found the leaflet adequate, that they understood the content or if further information was needed. Serious problems could follow if a parent with literacy difficulties is supplied with a leaflet about their child's medication without accompanying explanation. Parents with literacy difficulties can become expert at disguising their abilities, and verbal discussion should support the supply of all written information.

Seeking health information from the internet

The internet is a widely available, affordable and interactive multi-media source which is emerging as one of the most common ways children and young people

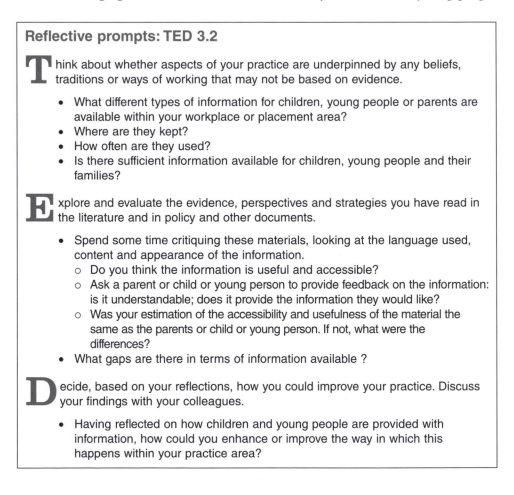

Reflective prompts: TED 3.2

Think about whether aspects of your practice are underpinned by any beliefs, traditions or ways of working that may not be based on evidence.

- What different types of information for children, young people or parents are available within your workplace or placement area?
- Where are they kept?
- How often are they used?
- Is there sufficient information available for children, young people and their families?

Explore and evaluate the evidence, perspectives and strategies you have read in the literature and in policy and other documents.

- Spend some time critiquing these materials, looking at the language used, content and appearance of the information.
  - Do you think the information is useful and accessible?
  - Ask a parent or child or young person to provide feedback on the information: is it understandable; does it provide the information they would like?
  - Was your estimation of the accessibility and usefulness of the material the same as the parents or child or young person. If not, what were the differences?
- What gaps are there in terms of information available ?

Decide, based on your reflections, how you could improve your practice. Discuss your findings with your colleagues.

- Having reflected on how children and young people are provided with information, how could you enhance or improve the way in which this happens within your practice area?

communicate socially (Stinson et al. 2012), with the majority of children and young people in countries such as the UK, USA and Australia having access to the internet either at school or at home (http://www.internetworldstats.com/stats. htm). Indeed, children's and young people's ways of accessing the internet are constantly changing, with more and more young people accessing information on mobile devices. The internet has been shown to be highly acceptable way for children and young people with health problems to access condition specific information (Stinson et al. 2010) and also as a way for children and young people to access general health information to support information received from health care professionals, school and family (Franck and Noble 2007). Information obtained over the internet has been used to provide self-management strategies relating to conditions such as asthma (Rikkers-Mutsaerts et al. 2012) and encopresis (Ritterband et al. 2003) with positive effect. The internet is also a valuable source of information for parents on their child's general health and behaviour (Bernhardt and Felter 2004; Khoo et al. 2008) or relating to specific health concerns (Oprescu et al. 2013; Sim et al. 2007), or acting as a source of support (Paterson et al. 2013; Stewart et al. 2011), especially for rare conditions where there is little information or support locally (Leonard et al. 2004; Oprescu et al. 2013).

The internet allows people to seek information on health questions which are perceived to be sensitive, embarrassing or awkward and which they may have otherwise struggled to share face to face with family, peers or health professionals. However, some information accessed on the internet can be inaccurate, incomplete, of poor quality (Fergie et al. 2012; Khoo et al. 2008), too difficult for children and young people to read (Stinson et al. 2011) or out of date (Franck and Noble 2007). The amount of information on the internet can also be overwhelming for parents and it can be hard and time consuming to judge the credibility and accuracy of the information (Stinson et al. 2012). Many health professionals can describe instances where parents have produced inaccurate information about their child's condition or treatment options gained from the internet; this can create difficulties. It could be argued that if health professionals provided parents with comprehensive information or guided them to information to help them develop their understanding, parents would feel less need to go in search of information on the internet.

Parents and young people can find the social support aspects of the internet useful, especially where discussion boards, chat rooms and social networking sites provide the opportunity to talk and share experiences with others who are not in their locality. This can help when children, young people or parents feel they are the only ones dealing with a certain condition or complications; people have described moments of revelation that it is 'not just them' on this illness journey. Young people may choose to seek factual information from health professionals and psychosocial information from the internet (Gray et al. 2005). Some information on the internet can be confusing and may rely heavily on textual sources of information. School-aged children recommend that health information on the internet targeted at their age group should be supported by games, animations and videos with minimal text (Franck and Noble

2007; Stinson et al. 2012). Young people have expressed a preference for internet health information to be gender specific (Franck and Noble 2007) and customised to the specific group accessing it. Although children and young people are often assumed to be more technologically competent than many adults, studies have shown that some children and young people can struggle with determining the credibility of information on the internet (Gray et al. 2005) and can have difficulty constructing effective search queries (Bilal and Kirby 2002).

Reflective prompts: TED 3.3

Think about whether aspects of your practice are underpinned by any beliefs, traditions or ways of working that may not be based on evidence.

- Think of a procedure which is conducted within your practice area. Note down the information and preparation a child usually receives before this is carried out.
- What are the advantages and disadvantages of the current preparation?
- What influences how this is done?
- How much time is taken in preparing a child for a procedure?
- Who does the preparation and who is the preparation focused on?
- How adequate do you think the information and preparation is?

Explore and evaluate the evidence, perspectives and strategies you have read in the literature and in policy and other documents.

- How could Alison (Jayden's mother) be engaged to help prepare Jayden for the procedure?
- What information or script could help Jayden prepare for his cannulation?
- How might this be different to a child going to their general practitioner or practice nurse for routine blood to be taken?

Decide, based on your reflections, how you could improve your practice. Discuss your findings with your colleagues.

- How has your approach to providing information *and* preparation to children and young people changed as a result of reading this chapter and doing this activity?
- How might you try and implement this change into practice?

Preparing children and young people for procedures, interventions and condition changes

Providing timely and appropriate information before medical procedures has many benefits for children, parents and health professionals (Jaaniste et al. 2007). Fear of the unknown, uncertainty and a lack of explanation about procedures is one of the main causes of anxiety and distress for children and parents before admission to hospital (Felder-Puig et al. 2003; Wollin et al. 2004). This distress can continue to be experienced for several weeks after surgery through increased pain, anxiety and maladaptive behaviours (Kain et al. 2007). Providing information and preparing children aims to reduce this anxiety and distress and therefore improve both the inpatient stay and also the child's recovery after surgery. There are many different pre-operative preparation programmes for children, young people and parents which have variable effects in reducing children's and parents' pre-operative anxiety and improving outcomes after surgery (O'Connor 2000). The pre-operative programmes being offered in many children's hospitals include the opportunity to visit wards, play with medical equipment, meet specialist nurses or attend pre-assessment clinics. The attendance of families at face-to-face pre-operative preparation visits can be minimal (Smith and Callery 2005), especially for those families who live a distance away from the hospital. Parents and their children are encouraged to access 'virtual visits' to hospital or preparation programmes which are available in the form of online links and videos. Much of the research relating to providing information and preparing children coming to hospital has focused on surgery and there has been less exploration of how children and young people are prepared for procedures such as blood tests, X-rays, immunisations and dressing changes. Therefore, much of the discussion in this following section relates to children and young people coming to hospital for surgery, but the principles discussed are relevant to children and young people undergoing any type of planned procedure.

Case study 3.2: Jayden

Changes in competence

Jayden was 3 the last time he had an injection. Alison (his mother) explains to the nurse how he got really upset when the nurse tried to explain before his injection what they were going to do. Jayden's grandma speaks over her daughter to say 'it is always best not to say too much, isn't it, otherwise kids just worry don't they'.

Jayden is now 8 years old and his understanding and experience of illness and health interventions as well as his cognitive ability will have changed since his previous experience.

It is not clearly known how information provision before medical procedures influences the experiences of children and young people and different theories suggest information and preparation have different effects. One theory (script theory) describes how information provided, particularly to younger children, can be constructed into an expected sequence of events of what a visit to the doctors looks like and this can help prepare children for certain procedures (Nelson and Gruendel 1981). An example of how simple information may be portrayed to a young child is highlighted in Figure 3.2; either the health professional or the

You can sit on mum's/dad's/other's knee or a chair while we ask you a few
questions about how you cut your knee and have a little look.

We will then get some medicine for you, like you have at home, or put some
special medicine on your knee to make sure that it is not hurting you.

Then after a little bit we will give it a little clean and use some special glue to stick
it back together so it can get better.

We will put a special plaster on it so that it stays clean.

Then you can go home.

Figure 3.2   Example of a script that could be used to prepare a young child for a
                  procedure

parent could use this script to prepare a young child who needs to have a cut/
laceration on their knee glued in an accident and emergency or a walk-in centre
following a fall.

Models which advocate children being prepared using scripts suggest that although
the information may provoke an initial anxiety in children, the information allows
them to rehearse thoughts and images of the upcoming procedure and as a result,
when the procedure comes they are less anxious (Jaaniste et al. 2007). The provision
of information and preparation allows children and young people to develop realistic
expectations of what will happen which reduces fear of the unknown and allows
there to be congruence between expectations and actual experience (Chen et al.
2000). The provision of information will be different depending on children's
previous medical encounters. Information provided to children who have previous
experience of procedures will build on their existing expectations and experiences
and their already constructed schemata or scripts for what they expect will happen
when they go to hospital.

Timing

Information provision should be timed so that children and young people have time
to develop an appropriate schemata or idea of what is going to happen to help them
prepare and rehearse coping strategies (Jaaniste et al. 2007). There is no clear guidance
as to how long before admission or a procedure children should be given information
and it can often be that information is delivered in small 'bite-size' chunks over a
period of time to allow children the opportunity to think through different aspects of
the information they receive and to ask questions. Younger children will not retain
information over a long period of time before a procedure and it is generally advised
that information is best provided a few days before an admission or procedure
(Jaaniste et al. 2007). Older children (aged 5–12 years old) have indicated that they

prefer to be told about hospitalisation as least a week before the event (Ross 1984). Giving children information too near to a procedure or admission can cause heightened anxiety (Kain et al. 1996), as they do not have time to process the information. Some parents may choose to not tell their children at all about an impending procedure, especially if their child has experienced distress having a procedure before, although this can compound the on-going and future distress of the child for subsequent procedures as they have not had the opportunity to develop a script of expectations and to focus on positive aspects of previous procedures (Jaaniste et al. 2007). The following quote is from a parent whose child was having a venous blood test, who withheld information from her child in order to prevent upset.

> When the doctor came in with the stuff I just said '(child's name) can you just sit on my knee' she sat on my knee and I said 'they just want to look at your hand darling it won't hurt, they're just going to have a quick look'. I didn't tell her what they were going to do. (Parent of child aged 3 years, Bray et al. 2012)

This 'glossing over the bad bits' by the parent was not recognised or challenged by the health professionals who came to do the test. Although the girl held her hand still, as soon as she felt the needle she became very upset and this may mean she will be less likely to offer her hand in the future.

The timing of information provision will depend on the age of the child and their cognitive development. If a child has just arrived in the clinic or ward for a procedure to be carried out their capacity to absorb, understand and process information may be less than when information is delivered at home before leaving for the hospital or clinic. Likewise, many parents will be able to recount stories of telling their child information which then led to a few days of difficult questions, excitement and altered behaviour, and sometimes, on reflection, parents may feel that it would have been better to have waited. However, all these reactions of children to information can be seen to be part of developing a script, with each question adding some context to what may happen, where and why. Due to decreasing amounts of time spent by children in acute care settings before surgery or procedures, there can be limited time for health professionals to spend with children preparing them for procedures (Ford et al. 2012). It may be that parents are left to carry out this role. However, it cannot be assumed that parents are willing or competent to take on this role. They may not know what information to give, or when it is best given and may not be able to answer their child's queries. The increasing use of day case surgery and short stays can mean that there is also less time for children to become accustomed to and familiar with the health care environment and the uniforms and equipment which dominate acute settings.

Content of preparation

Preparation for younger children may focus on concrete events such as what the room will look like, where the procedure will take place and who will be there.

Preparation and information for older children may concentrate on what they may feel and more detail on what will happen, with analogies being particularly useful, for example 'It will be like ... '. In all age groups the combination of procedural information (what health professionals will do) and sensory information (what the children will feel or experience during the procedure) is seen to be most effective (Jaaniste et al. 2007). Providing specific information can be problematic if parents do not have adequate knowledge themselves of what the procedure will involve, and they may even provide inaccurate information. The way information is presented is important. If information is presented in an unsuitable manner, for example using graphic procedural pictures (Jaaniste et al. 2007) or detailed verbal surgical explanation (Bray et al. 2012) pre-operative anxiety and distress may be increased.

As in work with adults, the provision of information to children has been shown to be influenced by whether children and young people are information seekers or information avoiders (Petersen and Toler 1986). Anyone who has worked with children will have witnessed children who want to watch their wound being stitched and ask lots of questions about what is happening compared to those who wish to bury their face and be distracted away from watching or thinking about it. There is more work to be done to determine the best way to prepare children based on their individual preferences for information.

Reflective prompts: TED 3.4

Think about whether aspects of your practice are underpinned by any beliefs, traditions or ways of working that may not be based on evidence.

- Think of a procedure which is conducted within your practice area. Note down the information and preparation a child normally receives before this is carried out.
- What are the advantages and disadvantages of current preparation?
- What influences how this is done?

Explore and evaluate the evidence, perspectives and strategies you have read in the literature and in policy and other documents.

- What information could help Jayden prepare for his cannulation?
- Write a script to help you communicate effectively with Jayden.
  - Revise the script so that you can communicate with a child younger and one older than Jayden.
- How might this be different to a child going to their general practitioner or practice nurse for routine blood to be taken?

Decide, based on your reflections, how you could improve your practice. Discuss your findings with your colleagues.

- How has your approach to providing information and preparation to children and young people changed as a result of reading this chapter and doing this activity?

Conclusion

Children and young people are competent reporters of their lives and health experiences. It is important for children and young people to have opportunities to gain and share information in a meaningful way in order for them to prepare themselves for procedures, interventions and the management of long-term conditions. Parents and health professionals should act as advocates to ensure that children and young people can access information. Withholding information or the (over)protection of children and young people from perceived harmful or anxiety-provoking information can result in trust with parents or health professionals being eroded and negative long-term outcomes. When provided with honest, appropriate written, verbal or online information children and young people can become active participants in health care decisions. Children and young people will have individual preferences and priorities in terms of information and these must be acknowledged and not subsumed within family or parental preferences.

References

Aronsson, K. and Rundstrom, B. (1989) 'Cats, dogs, and sweets in the clinical negotiation of reality: on politeness and coherence in pediatric discourse', *Language in Society*, 18(4): 483–504.

Beresford, B. and Sloper, P. (2003) 'Chronically ill adolescents' experiences of communicating with doctors: a qualitative study', *Journal of Adolescent Health*, 33(3): 172–179.

Bernhardt, J.M. and Felter, E.M. (2004) 'Online pediatric information seeking among mothers of young children: results from a qualitative study using focus groups', *Journal of Medical Internet Research*, 6(1): e7.

Bilal, D. and Kirby, J. (2002) 'Differences and similarities in information seeking: children and adults as web users', *Information Processing & Management*, 38(5): 649–670.

Bluebond-Langner, M. (1978) *The Private World of Dying Children*. Princeton: Princeton University Press.

Bray, L. (2010) 'The experiences of children, young people and their parents' of having and living with a continent stoma'. Unpublished PhD thesis.

Bray, L., Callery, P. and Kirk, S. (2012) 'A qualitative study of the pre-operative preparation of children, young people and their parents for planned continence surgery: experiences and expectations', *Journal of Clinical Nursing*, 21(13–14): 1964–1973.

Bristol Royal Infirmary Inquiry (2001) *The Report of the Public Inquiry into Children's Heart Surgery at the Bristol Royal Infirmary 1984–1995: Learning from Bristol*. Available at: http://webarchive.nationalarchives.gov.uk/20090811143745/http://www.bristol-inquiry.org.uk/final_report/report/index.htm (accessed 26/06/2013)

Bruera, E., Pituskin, E., Calder, K., Neumann, C.M. and Hanson, J. (1999) 'The addition of an audiocassette recording of a consultation to written recommendations for patients with advanced cancer', *Cancer*, 86(11): 2420–2425.

Cahill, P. and Papageorgiou, A. (2007) 'Triadic communication in the primary care paediatric consultation: a review of the literature', *The British Journal of General Practice*, 57(544): 904–911.

Callery, P. and Milnes, L. (2012) 'Communication between nurses, children and their parents in asthma review consultations', *Journal of Clinical Nursing*, 21(11–12): 1641–1650.

Carter, B. (2002) 'Chronic pain in childhood and the medical encounter: professional ventriloquism and hidden voices', *Qualitative Health Research*, 12 (1): 28–41.

Cegala, D.J., Coleman, M.T. and Turner, J.W. (1998) 'The development and partial assessment of the medical communication competence scale', *Health Communication*, 10(3): 261–288.

Chen, E., Joseph, M.H. and Zeltzer, L.K. (2000) 'Behavioral and cognitive interventions in the treatment of pain in children', *Pediatric Clinics of North America*, 47(3): 513–525.

Coyne, I. and Kirwan, L. (2012) 'Ascertaining children's wishes and feelings about hospital life', *Journal of Child Health Care*, 16(3): 293–304.

D'Alessandro, D.M., Kreiter, C.D., Kinzer, S.L. and Peterson, M.W. (2004) 'A randomized controlled trial of an information prescription for pediatric patient education on the internet', *Archives of Pediatrics & Adolescent Medicine*, 158(9): 857–862.

Department for Education and Skills and the Department of Health (2003) *Together from the Start – Practical Guidance for Professionals Working with Disabled Children (Birth to Third Birthday) and their Families*. London and Nottingham: Department for Education and Skills and the Department of Health.

Department of Health (2004) *National Service Framework for Children, Young People and Maternity Services*. London: DH.

Eden, O., Black, I. and Emery, A. (1993) 'The use of taped parental interviews to improve communication with childhood cancer families', *Pediatric Hematology-Oncology*, 10(2): 157–162.

Felder-Puig, R., Maksys, A., Noestlinger, C., Gadner, H., Stark, H., Pfluegler, A. and Topf, R. (2003) 'Using a children's book to prepare children and parents for elective ENT surgery: results of a randomized clinical trials', *International Journal of Pediatric Otorhinolaryngology*, 67(1): 35–41.

Fergie, G., Hunt, K. and Hilton, S. (2012) 'What young people want from health-related online resources: a focus group study', *Journal of Youth Studies*, 16(5): 579–596.

Ford, K., Courteney-Pratt, H. and Fitzgerald, M. (2012) 'Post-discharge experiences of children and their families following children's surgery', *Journal of Child Health Care*, 16(4): 320–30.

Franck, L.S. and Noble, G. (2007) 'Here's an idea: ask the users! Young people's views on navigation, design and content of a health information website', *Journal of Child Health Care*, 11(4): 287–297.

Gibson, F., Richardson, A., Hey, S., Horstman, M. and O'Leary, C. (2005) *Listening to Children and Young People with Cancer*. Final Report Submitted to Macmillan Cancer Support, London.

Gray, N.J., Klein, J.D., Noyce, P.R., Sesselberg, T.S. and Cantrill, J.A. (2005) 'The internet: a window on adolescent health literacy', *Journal of Adolescent Health*, 37(3): e1–243.

Jaaniste, T., Hayes, B. and Von Baeyer, C.L. (2007) 'Providing children with information about forthcoming medical procedures: a review and synthesis', *Clinical Psychology: Science and Practice*, 14(2): 124–143.

James, A. and Prout, A. (2004) *Constructing and Reconstructing Childhood: Contemporary Issues in the Sociological Study of Childhood*. Abingdon: Routledge.

Jurkovich, G.J., Pierce, B., Pananen, L. and Rivara, F.P. (2000) 'Giving bad news: the family perspective', *The Journal of Trauma and Acute Care Surgery*, 48(5): 865–873.

Kain, Z.N., Mayes, L.C., O'Connor, T.Z. and Cicchetti, D.V. (1996) 'Preoperative anxiety in children: predictors and outcomes', *Archives of Pediatrics & Adolescent Medicine*, 150(12): 1238–1245.

Kain, Z.N., Caldwell-Andrews, A.A., Mayes, L.C., Weinberg, M.E., Wang, S., MacLaren, J.E. and Blount, R.L. (2007) 'Family-centered preparation for surgery improves perioperative outcomes in children: a randomized controlled trial', *Anesthesiology*, 106(1): 65–74.

Khoo, K., Bolt, P., Babl, F.E., Jury, S. and Goldman, R.D. (2008) 'Health information seeking by parents in the internet age', *Journal of Paediatrics and Child Health*, 44(7–8): 419–423.

Kreicbergs, U., Valdimarsdóttir, U., Onelöv, E., Henter, J. and Steineck, G. (2004) 'Talking about death with children who have severe malignant disease', *New England Journal of Medicine*, 351(12): 1175–1186.

Lambert, S.D. and Loiselle, C.G. (2007) 'Health information-seeking behavior', *Qualitative Health Research*, 17(8): 1006–1019.

Lambert, V., Glacken, M. and McCarron, M. (2008) '"Visible-ness": the nature of communication for children admitted to a specialist children's hospital in the Republic of Ireland', *Journal of Clinical Nursing*, 17(23): 3092–3102.

Leonard, H., Slack-Smith, L., Phillips, T., Richardson, S., D'Orsogna, L. and Mulroy, S. (2004) 'How can the internet help parents of children with rare neurologic disorders?', *Journal of Child Neurology*, 19(11): 902–907.

Levetown, M. (2008) 'Communicating with children and families: from everyday interactions to skill in conveying distressing information', *Pediatrics*, 121(5): 1441–1460.

Lewis, C., Skirton, H. and Jones, R. (2012) 'Development of an evidence-based information booklet to support parents of children without a diagnosis', *Journal of Genetic Counseling*, 21(6): 854–861.

McGuigan, F. and Salmon, K. (2005) 'Pre-event discussion and recall of a novel event: How are children best prepared?', *Journal of Experimental Child Psychology*, 91(4): 342–366.

Nelson, K & Gruendel, J.M (1981) 'Generalised representations, basic building blocks of cognitive development'. In M.E Lamb and A.L. Brown (eds) *Advances in Developmental Psychology. Vol 1*. Hillsdale, NJ: Erlbaum.

Nelson, K. and Gruendel, J. (1989) 'Children's scripts', in K. Nelson (ed.) *Event Knowledge: Structure and Function in Development*. Mahwah, NJ: Lawrence Erlbaum Associates, pp. 21–46.

Nova, C., Vegni, E. and Moja, E.A. (2005) 'The physician-patient-parent communication: a qualitative perspective on the child's contribution', *Patient Education and Counseling*, 58(3): 327–333.

O'Conner-Van, S. (2000) 'Preparing children for surgery – an integrative research review', *AORN Journal*, 71(2): 334–343.

Oprescu, F., Campo, S., Lowe, J., Andsager, J. and Morcuende, J.A. (2013) 'Online information exchanges for parents of children with a rare health condition: key findings from an online support community', *Journal of Medical Internet Research*, 15(1): e16.

Paterson, B.L., Brewer, J. and Stamler, L.L. (2012) 'Engagement of parents in on-line social support interventions', *Journal of Pediatric Nursing*, 28(2): 114–124.

Perrin, E.C., Lewkowicz, C. and Young, M.H (2000) 'Shared vision: concordance among fathers, mothers, and pediatricians about unmet needs of children with chronic health conditions', *Pediatrics*, 105 (Supp 2): 277–85.

Peterson, L. and Toler, S.M. (1986) 'An information seeking disposition in child surgery patients', *Health Psychology*, 5(4): 343–358.

Rikkers-Mutsaerts, E.R.V.M., Winters A.E., Bakker, M.J., van Stel, H.F., van der Meer, H.F., de Jongste, J.C. and Sont, J.K. (2012) 'Internet-based self-management compared with usual care in adolescents with asthma: A randomized controlled trial', *Pediatric Pulmonology*, 47(12): 1170–79.

Ritterband, L.M., Cox, D.J., Walker, L.S., Kovatchev, B., McKnight, L., Patel, K., Borowitz, S. and Sutphen, J. (2003) 'An internet intervention as adjunctive therapy for pediatric enco-presis', *Journal of Consulting and Clinical Psychology*, 71(5): 910–917.

Ross, S.A. (1984) 'Impending hospitalization: timing of preparation for the school-aged child', *Children's Health Care*, 12(4): 187–189.

Rouck, S. and Leys, M. (2012) 'Illness trajectory and internet as a health information and communication channel used by parents of infants admitted to a neonatal intensive care unit', *Journal of Advanced Nursing*, 69(7): 1489–1499.

Sanders, C., Carter, B. and Goodacre, L. (2011) 'Searching for harmony: parents' narratives about their child's genital ambiguity and reconstructive genital surgeries in childhood', *Journal of Advanced Nursing*, 67(10): 2220–2230.

Savage, E. and Callery, P. (2007) 'Clinic consultations with children and parents on the dietary management of cystic fibrosis', *Social Science & Medicine*, 64(2): 363–374.

Scott, S., Hartling, L., O'Leary, K.A., Archibald, M. and Klassen, T.P. (2012) 'Stories – a novel approach to transfer complex health information to parents: a qualitative study', *Arts & Health: An International Journal for Research, Policy and Practice*, 4(2): 162–173.

Sim, N.Z., Kitteringham, L., Spitz, L., Pierro, A., Kiely, E., Drake, D. and Curry, J. (2007) 'Information on the world wide web – how useful is it for parents?', *Journal of Pediatric Surgery*, 42(2): 305–312.

Smith, L. and Callery, P. (2005) 'Children's accounts of their preoperative information needs', *Journal of Clinical Nursing*, 14(2): 230–238.

Stewart, M., Letourneau, N., Masuda, J.R., Anderson, S. and McGhan, S. (2011) 'Online solutions to support needs and preferences of parents of children with asthma and allergies', *Journal of Family Nursing*, 17(3): 357–379.

Stinson, J.N., Toomey, P.C., Stevens, B.J., Kagan, S., Duffy, C.M., Huber, A., Malleson, P., McGrath, P.J., Yeung, R.S. and Feldman, B.M. (2008) 'Asking the experts: exploring the self-management needs of adolescents with arthritis', *Arthritis Care & Research*, 59(1): 65–72.

Stinson, J.N., McGrath, P.J. Hodnett, E.D., Feldman, B.M., Duffy, C.M., Huber, A.M., Tucker, L.B., Hetherington, R., Tse, S.M.L., Spiegel, L.R., Campillo, S., Gill, N.K and White. M.E (2010) 'An internet-based self-management program with telephone support for adolescents with arthritis: a pilot randomized controlled trial', *The Journal of Rheumatology*, 37(9): 1944–52.

Stinson, J.N., White, M., Breakey, V., Chong A.L., Mak, I., Koekebakker Low, K. and Koekebakker Low, A. (2011) 'Perspectives on quality and content of information on the internet for adolescents with cancer', *Pediatric Blood & Cancer*, 57(1): 97–104.

Stinson, J.N., Feldman, B.M., Duffy, C.M., Huber, A.M., Tucker, L.B., McGrath, P.J., Shirley, M., Hetherington, R., Spiegel, L.R. and Campillo, S. (2012) 'Jointly managing arthritis: information needs of children with juvenile idiopathic arthritis (JIA) and their parents', *Journal of Child Health Care*, 16(2): 124–140.

Tates, K. and Meeuwesen, L. (2000) '"Let Mum have her say": turn taking in doctor–parent–child communication', *Patient Education and Counselling*, 151–62.

Tates, K. and Meeuwesen, L. (2001) 'Doctor–parent–child communication: a (re)view of the literature', *Social Science & Medicine*, 52(6): 839–851.

Trollvik, A., Ringsberg, K.C. and Silén, C. (2013) 'Children's experiences of a participation approach to asthma education', *Journal of Clinical Nursing*, 22 (7–8): 996–1004.

UN General Assembly (1989) *Convention on the Rights of the Child*. Geneva: United Nations.

van Dulmen, A.M. (1998) 'Children's contributions to pediatric outpatient encounters', *Pediatrics*, 102(3): 563–568.

Wollin, S.R., Plummer, J.L., Owen, H., Hawkins, R.M., Materazzo, F. and Morrison, V. (2004) 'Anxiety in children having elective surgery', *Journal of Pediatric Nursing*, 19(2): 128–132.

Young, B., Dixon-Woods, M., Windridge, K.C. and Heney, D. (2003) 'Managing communication with young people who have a potentially life threatening chronic illness: qualitative study of patients and parents', *British Medical Journal*, 326(7384): 305.

Chapter 4

Children and Young People Having Choices and Making Health Decisions

Key points

- Children and young people can be excluded from making decisions about their health care and treatment based on misconceptions that they lack the ability to understand difficult medical information.
- Professionals need to communicate with children, young people and their parents to find out how involved they want to be in decisions and choices about their care.
- If children and young people are not competent to provide consent for treatment or surgery they should be provided with the opportunity to express an opinion about their care and for this to be listened to.
- Factors which can influence children's and young people's ability to make decisions include age, previous illness, health care or decision-making experience, dynamics within a family and the actions and inactions of professionals.

Key theories and concepts explored in this chapter are competence, consent, assent, decision making and autonomy.

Case study 4.1: Rachel

Setting the scene

Rachel is a 14-year-old who has lived with a long-term continence condition since birth. She had an operation when she was 8 years old to form a continent channel into her bowel into which she is prescribed a daily saline washout in order for her to manage her constipation and remain continent. The regime requires her to spend an hour each evening in the bathroom, which although Rachel feels is 'a pain' means she no longer soils at school, something which she hated and resulted in teasing by a group of girls from her class. The bowel washout increasingly interferes with her ability to socialise with her friends. She now also has a boyfriend. Rachel lives with her mum and dad who have always supported her in independently

(Continued)

> *(Continued)*
>
> carrying out her regime. Her mum and dad have noticed and become concerned that she has not been doing her washout regime every night. When they confront her Rachel states 'I'm not doing the washouts any longer, they take too much time and I'm doing okay. I'm not constipated'. Her parents are concerned as her appetite has decreased and they insist that she does her washout. When they attend their regular outpatient appointment there is obvious tension when Rachel says 'she wants to go in on her own' to see the medical and nursing staff without her parents.

Introduction

This chapter will discuss the complexity which can surround making health decisions and choices with children and young people and their parents. The chapter aims to debate the more day-to-day issues involved in helping children and young people to make meaningful choices and decisions in relation to their health and health care, sometimes when these are not even recognised as being choices and decisions. This discussion will not focus on the difficult and relatively rare legal cases within health care where courts have to make decisions on the rights of children in relation to very complex issues such as donating organs or withdrawing and withholding treatment as there are texts which dedicate themselves to these circumstances.

Making decisions

In order to discuss children and young people making decisions and choices in health care it is important to briefly outline the concepts and terms used, many of which stem from literature addressing adult decision making.

Making decisions as an adult

The ability to make a decision as an adult is influenced by the individual's competency (capacity) and the opportunity to make a voluntary choice based on having appropriate information (Applebaum 2007). Competency is related to a person's cognitive development, the type of decision being made and the context in which the decision is made (Ross 1998). Adults make decisions all the time, often without too much deliberation, such as what to have for breakfast, for example weighing up between a healthy cereal or a convenient ready-made breakfast bar. The process used to make all decisions, even simple ones, has been differentiated into distinct steps:

1. Identification of possible decision options (cereal or bar);
2. Identification of possible risks and benefits associated with each option (healthier cereal, higher salt and sugar levels in bar);

3. Evaluation of the desirability of each consequence (bar more convenient and late for work but may lead to snacking later in the day); and

4. Assessment of the likelihood of each consequence and combination of the above information using some decision-making rule such as identifying the best option or course of action (Beyth-Marom et al. 1993).

Adults are practised in making decisions, the process often happens quickly and without too much thought, hopefully with the best course of action being chosen.

Making health and treatment decisions tends to be more complicated than day-to-day choices such as what to eat for breakfast or how to spend a day off work. Even when adults have competency they may wish to be involved in health care decisions in different ways, with some people keen to take a lead on making decisions regarding their care while some may prefer to hand over the responsibility for decisions to their health care team (Levinson et al. 2005). There are certain instances where adults may not be deemed able to make a decision, such as when a person has a severe debilitating neurological condition. In cases where there is a lack of competency, it may be that shared decision making can be promoted or responsibility for decisions needs to be handed to a substitute decision-maker or, in cases of emergency treatment, to a medical team. The traditional and dominant view in many health care settings is that children are not competent to make decisions about their health care and their substitute decision maker will in most cases be their parent.

Making decisions as a parent

Legally parents have the responsibility for making decisions on behalf of their children, therefore it is important that parents themselves are competent and have adequate information to make informed decisions (Ellison 2007). This may seem straightforward but often decisions have to be made which involve children experiencing pain, discomfort or unpleasant procedures. Making a decision to subject their child to a painful procedure can be difficult and upsetting for parents and seeing their child upset or seriously ill can negatively influence parents' ability to process complicated information and make appropriate decisions (Ellison 2007). In these instances parents still need to weigh up risks versus benefits and the consequences of their decisions, just as they would when making minor day-to-day decisions, but health decisions in stressful circumstances can be very difficult and different to their experience in making everyday decisions. Parents of children with cancer have expressed how they felt a lack of control over decisions during stressful times (Levi et al. 2000) and felt they needed more time to consider treatment options (Kilicarslan-Toruner and Akgun-Citak 2013; McKenna et al. 2010). The anxiety and stress parents experience in making decisions on behalf of their child is not just in cases of life limiting illnesses; parents also find consenting for planned surgery daunting (Bray et al. 2012; Pfeil 2011) and making decisions about embarking on new treatments (Sanders and Bray 2013).

Evidence suggests a mismatch between health professionals' and parents' expectations of their roles in making decisions (Fiks et al. 2011). There is often no opportunity for lengthy open dialogue about what decisions are being made within an emergency situation, but in planned treatment discussions, parents should have the opportunity to express their anxiety and preferred role in making decisions.

As infants become children and then young people, the parental role changes from making decisions and choices *for* their child to facilitating their child's involvement in making decisions. Although parents identify that it is important for their child to be involved in decisions, they can have concerns that their child may choose the 'wrong' decision or that being asked to make treatment decisions is too great a burden for their child (Coyne 2006a). There can be a difficult balancing act between protecting children from upsetting information and difficult choices and allowing them the opportunity to participate in making choices and decisions (Bray et al. 2012; Coyne and Harder 2011).

Unfortunately, excluding children from participating in making decisions can actually increase their fear and bewilderment (Alderson 1993). Yet children are often far more aware of what is going on than they are given credit for and attuned to when they are excluded from 'something that is going on'. Parents may need encouragement from health professionals to have the confidence to allow their child to be involved in decisions and choices about their health care (Alderson and Montgomery 1996). Parents in a stressful situation can act in accordance with their own interests or the interests of professionals rather than taking the side of their child (Leikin 1989). In a study exploring how children and young people are held for clinical procedures, parents and health professionals were observed to frequently 'join forces' in an unspoken pact to hold children in order for a procedure to be completed despite the child being distressed (Bray et al. 2012). In these situations parents may be overwhelmed and frightened themselves and not aware that there might be other alternatives to forcefully holding their child. Parents in these circumstances could be seen as unable to act as an advocate for their child. In these cases it should be health professionals who act as advocates for the child's best interests and make sure that children are given the opportunity to have a voice (Runeson et al. 2001). Health professionals should feel prepared to question practice and take action, if necessary, to ensure children and young people are given choices and their voice does not get drowned out by those of adults.

Children and young people making medical decisions

International guidance (UN General Assembly 1989) identifies children and young people (those under 18 years of age) as individuals in their own right, with their own rights, specifically their right to participate in decisions that affect them. This is supported by society in general increasingly recognising the ability of children and young people to report on their own lives and rely less on parents or professionals to speak *for* them (James and Prout 2004). There are international debates about the rights of children and young people to make medical decisions, and there are national differences in how guidance is interpreted. In Sweden the duty of parents and society is promoted over the rights of the child (Mårtenson and Fägerskiöld 2008), whereas legislation in Canada (Health Care Concern Act 1996) focuses on individuals (regardless of age) being capable of consenting to or refusing medical treatment unless they are found incapable (Geist and Opler 2010).

Although there is a clearly specified legal age of majority (which differs across countries from 16 to 21 years of age), a young person does not suddenly wake up on their sixteenth or eighteenth birthday having developed competency overnight and it can be difficult to pinpoint an age when a young person is competent to make treatment decisions. There may be some instances where young people need to make unsupervised decisions under the age of 16 years. In England and Wales, common law, often referred to as Gillick competence, is used to judge if a young person under the age of 16 years is competent to make medical decisions (Wheeler 2006). Although this legal ruling was initially concerned with the prescription of contraception, the term Gillick competence is now used in a broader sense relating to young people seeking or receiving medical care or treatment without their parents' consent. The ruling of Gillick competence is now recognised or referred to in legal guidance outside the UK, for example in Australia, Canada and New Zealand. The adaptation of this ruling into professional regulations tends to focus on the intellectual understanding and cognitive competence of children and young people and fails to acknowledge children's and young people's developing ability to place information in a wider social context and understand the moral implications of their decisions and the impact they may have on the family (Ellison 2007).

Although there are national, individual and situational differences which influence how young people are involved in health and treatment decisions and choices, guidance is more prescriptive regarding children's and young people's involvement in research. Commonly children have a higher involvement and

---

Reflective prompts: TED 4.1

Think about whether aspects of your practice are underpinned by any beliefs, traditions or ways of working that may not be based on evidence.

- Thinking about Rachel, do you think she is old enough to make decisions about the management of her condition?
- From your experience, can you think what may influence how you involve children and young people in making decisions or choices?

Explore and evaluate the evidence, perspectives and strategies you have read in the literature and in policy and other documents.

- What literature has informed your thinking?
- What documents within your workplace inform how children and young people are supported to make decisions or have a voice?

Decide, based on your reflections, how you could improve your practice. Discuss your findings with your colleagues.

- How could Rachel's ability to make decisions be judged and supported?
- Having reflected on how children and young people are facilitated to be involved in decisions and choices, how could you enhance or improve the way in which this happens within your practice area?

recognition of their decisions as a research participant than they do as a patient (Alderson 2007). This is because research involvement is seen as an addition to standard medical care, so therefore it is often easier for children, young people and parents to decide whether or not to take part. Parents cannot over-ride children's decisions relating to research involvement. Even very young children who refuse or resist involvement in research cannot be enrolled into a study (RCPCH 2000, in Alderson 2007).There are variations in the consent procedures, for example clinical trials involving children and young people (aged less than 18 years of age) legally have to seek parental consent, yet this may not be the case for other non-therapeutic research within health and social care which is perceived to be associated with less risk to participants (National Health and Medical Research Council 2013).

Characteristics influencing children's and young people's competency

Working with children and young people is a complex and rewarding experience and involving children and young people in their health care presents many different challenges and opportunities. As discussed in the previous section, every child is an individual with different competencies and abilities in making medical decisions. It can be very subjective and difficult to determine whether a young person has the ability to give consent to their medical treatment or care. Assent is a concept used with children who do not have the ability to provide consent and this will be discussed in more detail later in the chapter. Judgement of capacity is often assumed to lie with the health professional, but it may be best made within an on-going social group such as the family unit (Children's Hospitals Australasia 2010) rather than with a professional who may have limited knowledge of the young person. This may prove more challenging for children and young people who are in care and have had a limited opportunity to build up relationships with a close social group. These children and young people could be viewed as particularly vulnerable and are often reliant on professionals to make decisions with them in the absence of a permanent family group. It can also be problematic when there are competing agendas within a family group, especially when these are not expressed but run as an undercurrent during consultations. It may feel awkward, but it is important for professionals to encourage an open dialogue when decisions and choices are being made, and ensure that all family members have the opportunity to discuss their individual thoughts, beliefs, misconceptions or concerns.

Judging the competency of children or young people to make decisions or choices is subjective and influenced by many characteristics including the education of the child or young person, the protest of the child (Runeson et al. 2001), the attitudes of health professionals (Runeson et al. 2001) and the family context. The following sections discuss the two most commonly stated characteristics which can influence competency: age (Runeson et al. 2001) and previous illness experience (Alderson 1993; Crisp et al. 1996).

Age

It is commonly thought that age is the most important factor which determines children's and young people's understanding and competence. The ages of 7 to 11 years are frequently linked to attaining levels of competence, based on Piaget's theories, developed from the 1920s (Piaget 1924). At these ages, children are seen to change their understanding of illness; their views seem to be less concrete, less egocentric and their decisions are less likely to be influenced by others (Crisp et al. 1996). Children aged 7–11 years are seen as being capable of making increasingly independent choices, which consider the impact that their decisions will have on other people as well as on themselves. These prescriptive ages are still used to inform the provision of information and the involvement of children and young people in health choices and decisions. This is despite more recent research in which children and young people have displayed higher levels of competence and decision-making abilities than previously thought (Alderson 2007; Weithorn and Campbell 1982). The assessment of competence has been based on children and young people being exposed to hypothetical health situations or using children's reading ability (Billick et al. 1998; McAliley et al. 2000). Health choices and decisions are commonly more complicated and multi-dimensional than the single decision-tasks which have been used to determine the competency of children and young people.

Common sense dictates that a 2-year-old will be less able to make decisions about their care than a 12-year-old. Relying on age as a single determinant of competence becomes more problematic when a 6-year-old demonstrates through clear speech a willingness and understanding of relevant health choices and a 9-year-old does not become engaged in a consultation and looks blank when asked what they think. Previous theories of age-related competence would assume the 9-year-old has more competence than the 6-year-old. Likewise the quietness of the 9-year-old does not necessarily signify a lack of understanding but may be linked to an unfamiliar environment or an overzealous parent. This emphasises the importance of considering each child as an individual and not relying on age as the main indicator of competence (Halpern-Felsher and Cauffman 2001). Although some professional guidance still continues to quote age as a primary determinant of competence (Every Child Matters 2006 – in Alderson 2007), the recently published *Charter on the Rights of Children and Young People in Health Care Services in Australia* (2010) refers instead to children's and young peoples' experience and individual situations rather than age.

Experience

It is increasingly recognised that children's understanding and competence can depend far more on their experience than their age or ability (Alderson 2007: 2278). Many children and young people with congenital conditions, or who have long-term conditions, have extensive experience of their health needs and treatment and also of the systems and environment in which they receive care. This experience can often be gained over many years and they can become more informed than an adult experiencing their first acute illness episode.

Case study 4.2: Rachel

Familiarity and distance

Rachel has been involved in interactions with different professionals both within health contexts and in school regarding the management of her condition. She is familiar with clinic settings, inpatient wards and the language, terminology and dialogue used by professionals. As such she may be more able to be involved in discussions than another 14-year-old or even 16-year-old who has had no previous health care experience and who is anxious about being in an unfamiliar health environment. Established relationships with clinicians can be both enabling and disabling. Despite experience and familiarity within the health context and her clinical team, Rachel may feel less able to discuss her changing attitude with doctors and nurses she has known since she was a child.

Although it is important to acknowledge experience as a factor which can impact on competence, it should not be assumed that children or young people with long-term illnesses will *always* be more knowledgeable and competent to be involved in decisions than their counterparts with less experience. Children's and young peoples' experience of health services and their illness or condition does not always make them more able or willing to participate in the communication or decision-making processes (Bray et al. 2012; Lambert et al. 2008). One group of children and young people undergoing planned continence surgery who had experienced high levels of contact with health professionals, often since birth, reported low levels of involvement or understanding of information relating to their planned surgical procedure (Bray et al. 2012). It may also be the case that children and young people who demonstrate confidence and competence in relation to one aspect of their lives, such as the management of their diabetes, would become upset and unable to express an opinion when involved in an accident requiring some sutures within an emergency department, where they are unfamiliar with the environment and the health professionals working there. The influence of experience on understanding and competence is likely to be more complex than often implied. Work investigating the illness understanding of children and young people with long-term conditions compared to children and young people with minor complaints, demonstrated that previous experiences of illness aided understanding in children aged 7–10, but not those aged under and above this age group (Crisp et al. 1996). This work points to there being a relationship between age *and* experience and both need to be considered when engaging with children and young people. The factors which can influence children's and young people's competence to make decisions are illustrated in Figure 4.1.

Presence of parents and family dynamics

The section above has discussed the legal rulings which underpin children and young people making decisions within health care and the literature exploring

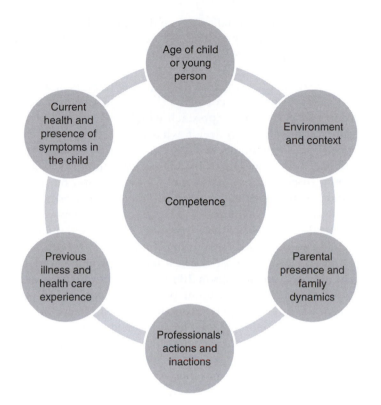

Figure 4.1   Factors which influence children's and young people's competence in making decisions

competence. The concept of competence to make decisions cannot be discussed without reference to autonomy and how children and young people are afforded the ability to make their *own* decisions and choices. Autonomy refers to a person having the power to make a free choice unconstrained by external agencies (Beauchamp and Childress 2001). Autonomy is a fundamental part of a person being able to provide consent for treatment and a child's autonomy is not an all or nothing concept, it will change and grow as the child matures (Runeson et al. 2002). Autonomy can have different interpretations within different cultures, and autonomy within some Eastern countries extends wider than an individual so that the family unit becomes the decision-making unit; maintaining family harmony has a high priority over individual preference (Lin et al. 2013).

As discussed previously it is unlikely that children or young people will be involved in making decisions or choices without the presence of their parents, carers or wider family; this presence can influence their ability to make decisions in a positive, neutral or negative way. Children can feel reassured and supported by the presence of their parents (especially their mothers), and have indicated how they can rely on them to be their voice within acute health settings (Livesley and Long 2013). When children's or young people's choices or decisions do not conform to those made by parents or health professionals then they may be labelled as non-compliant or non-concordant. It is challenging when children and young people are given the opportunity to make choices or decisions and the decisions made are different to what is perceived as best by the adults surrounding the child or young person.

In most cases where there is difficulty in children, young people, parents and/or health professionals agreeing to a course of clinical treatment or action, negotiation can result in consensus on an approach which best suits those involved. The principle which is applied to help decide what should happen when there is ongoing conflict between the opinions of children, young people, their parents or the health professional is the principle of the child's 'best interests'. The best interest principle is drawn from Article 3 (1) of the UN Convention on the Rights of the Child (1991) and is often given more weight than other articles which identify the rights of children to express their views and be afforded the opportunity to develop autonomy. The legal judgement of 'best interests' is not based on an objective ruling or criteria and can be a subjective ruling (Baines 2010). Both parents and the courts in England and Wales can use the best interest principle to defeat a competent child's refusal of treatment (Ellison 2007). This is not the case in all countries, and, for example, Swedish courts cannot pass judgement on individual cases of medical treatment (Mårtenson and Fägerskiöld 2008). There are discrepancies within the current legislation, where the legal framework allows young people to consent to care but not to refuse it when a doctor has decided it is in the young person's best interests.

As discussed within the chapter on family-centred care the different agendas of members within a family must also be considered when the best interest principle is being applied. Parents of children who are near the end of their life can sometimes make decisions to continue care beyond the child's best interests through their feelings of hope that 'something else can be done' to prolong their child's life (Baines 2010). Conversations to withdraw care can be challenging and emotionally charged. Also controversial are cases involving parental consent for children having cosmetic procedures (for example, prominent ears, removal of birthmarks) (Leshin 2000) or gender assignment (Sanders et al. 2012). These procedures can be viewed as being carried out to remove a child's differences and for them to conform to what is deemed by society and parents as acceptable (Hodges et al. 2002). Parents can be caught between wanting their child to appear 'normal' to peers and society and electing for their child to undergo a procedure which the child may not choose to have now or in the future.

As discussed in previous chapters, the delivery of care is moving away from a traditional paternalistic model (where health professionals take an authoritative role with little input from the patient) towards a more consultative and partnership approach which acknowledges the autonomy of a patient. Health professionals and patients should work together to reach a decision in a shared approach (Knopf et al. 2008) which recognises the expertise of both the professional and patient. This shared approach can become more complex where the relationship is not dyadic (two-way) between an adult patient and health professional, but is more triadic (three way) between the child or young person, parent and health professional. The dominance of adult voices (professionals and parents) within these consultations can lead to children and young people being marginalised, with health professionals directing their discussion of condition information and treatment choices to parents (Coyne 2006c; Ford 2010; Tates and Meeuwesen 2001). This, often unintentional exclusion, can impact on children's and young people's opportunities to gain experience in making decisions in a supportive environment. Children and young people have described instances where they were encouraged to make a decision which in principle had already been made by the adults in their lives (Bray et al. 2012), sometimes by parents or professionals making one option seem unattractive in an attempt to persuade them to choose what was deemed to be the 'right' choice (Miller 2009). In the following example a mother of an 11-year-old encouraged her daughter to make the decision about undergoing surgery for a long-term condition, even though this was the expected choice.

> At the end of the day I made her (daughter) make that decision after all, it was her that was having it and it was her body that it was getting done to. So it was alright for me to say 'yes, I want her to have it done' but what about her, it's her body. (Alice's mother) (Bray 2010: 129)

It can be hard in these instances for children and young people to question or 'go against' the perceived wisdom of the adults around them, or for their engagement in decisions to be meaningful and centred on their wishes. In contrast to reports of negative experiences, there are examples of parents acknowledging how consultations with professionals can pick up information from their children beyond what has been shared with them. There are also accounts from professionals which highlight how they work hard to ensure that the child is 'brought into' the consultation, even when the child's attitude is that 'they are here to see my mum' (Callery and Milnes 2012).

Young people are most frequently seen with their parents both within acute and primary care (Rutishauser et al. 2003), unless the young people have accessed a service independently, for example a sexual health clinic. Many young people with long-term conditions are transferred to adult provision, where, without adequate preparation, they may suddenly find themselves solely responsible for their care and health choices with minimal previous opportunity to practise these skills. It is being increasingly suggested that young people should be provided with the opportunity to have consultations with health professionals on their own without the presence of their parent (Rutishauser et al. 2003), giving them the opportunity to develop skills in order to participate in medical encounters when transferred to adult health care provision. It is important that in these instances, professionals do not fill the role of proxy parent for these young people. When faced with an apparently apathetic or apprehensive adolescent the professionals should not end up taking the lead in making decisions *for* the young people rather than spending time to allow the young people to become accustomed to receiving, sharing and giving information in an exchange which supports them to make decisions.

Involving children and young people in making choices and decisions

Although professionals are increasingly encouraged to involve children and young people in making decisions about their lives and health care, children and young people should also have the choice to actively decline being involved in making decisions. Children and young people have consistently shown a desire to be involved in decisions and choices relating to their care (Angst and Deatrick 1996; Bray et al. 2012; Dovey-Pearce at al. 2005), but may also choose not to be involved at other times (Coad and Houston 2007) or not take full responsibility for decision making (Boylan 2004). It is important that this is an active choice expressed and acknowledged and not a default mechanism used by adults to exclude children from the process. Children and young people may need more support to make decisions when the decision is bigger than others or when they have more severe symptoms and are more unwell (Miller 2009). It is important not to assume that children or young people either do or do not want to be involved in making decisions and choices about their care. Professionals should try and find out on an individual basis if a child or young person wants to participate and to what extent (Hallström and Elander 2004).

Children and young people with long-term or chronic conditions such as asthma or diabetes will make different decisions in different ways to those experiencing a one-off incident of acute illness. Decisions and choices about long-term illness or condition management are not only made within the health care environment (primary care and hospitals) but between children, young people and their families at home, school and in the workplace. There is little known about how these day-to-day decisions are made within these informal environments, although children who participate in decisions within the home and whose views are listened to and respected within this environment, may be better equipped to take part in more serious discussions within a health care context (Hallström and Elander 2004). An 11-year-old boy discussing the day-to-day decisions he makes regarding choices in his life (both condition-specific and everyday), revealed how he was 'allowed' to choose what he did when he got home after school, but was limited in what else he was 'allowed to decide' (Figure 4.2) (Bray 2010).

Management of conditions and decisions to take medications such as inhalers or injecting insulin are often not purely made according to symptoms or the prevention of symptoms (Meng and McConnell 2002) but can also be influenced by the perceived need to appear normal or to conceal the illness from peers, the degree of parental support and the need to reduce the disruptions to daily life. Young people can start to question how their regime influences and sometimes limits their social interaction and can make decisions and choices to try and reduce the impact their condition management regime has on their peer interaction (Atkin and Ahmad 2000). In many cases young people are seen as non-concordant when they do not follow the prescribed medical regime, although there is increasing discussion that decisions to alter regimes to adapt management into everyday life should be viewed less as not complying to medical regimens, but as recognising the expertise often built up by young people in managing their own conditions.

	What time I get up	What I wear for school	What I do after school	What time I do my catheter	Where I do my catheter
ME			✓		
MUM	✓	✓	✓	✓	✓
OTHER					✓

Figure 4.2 Choices and decisions of a young person managing a long-term continence condition

---

Case study 4.3: Rachel

Working together and fostering independence

Rachel's parents were happy to encourage and support Rachel in the independent management of her condition as long as she was following the agreed course of action of the professionals. When Rachel starts to make decisions regarding her condition management which do not 'fit' with the prescribed regime, she is considered to be not adhering to what is best for her health. Discussions and conflict within the family focus on what can be done to encourage her to continue with the prescribed regime. There is less discussion around what influences Rachel's decision to alter the way she manages her condition.

The developing ability of children and young people to make decisions and choices in the management of their condition is not always recognised by parents, who have often had sole responsibility for managing the long-term illness or condition (Bray et al. 2013). It can be hard for established roles and responsibilities to change within a family, and for parents to 'let go' of their ingrained caring and management activities. The tensions linked to young people exerting greater control over their lives are an everyday part of being a parent, but can be complicated by the presence of a long-term condition.

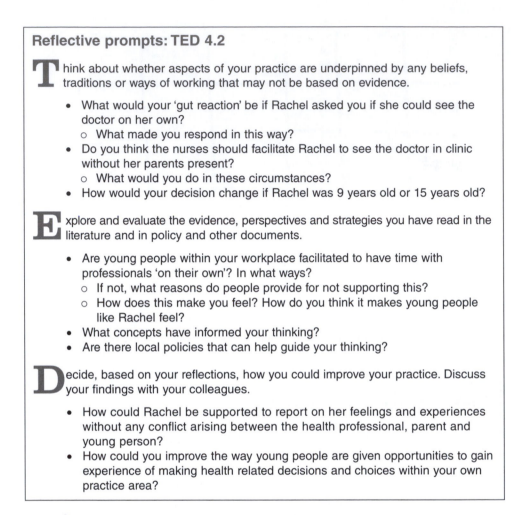

Children and young people making their own choices

Much of the dialogue regarding children's and young people's involvement in decisions focuses on planned consent for treatments such as surgery, medication regimes or other distinct interventions or procedures. There is less discussion on the nature of assent and on involving children and young people in more minor choices and decisions about their care. The concept of children providing assent is used in relation to involvement in research (Baines 2011; Bray 2007; Ford et al. 2007) and end of life care (Hinds et al. 2005; Kunin 1997) and less within day-to-day medical and nursing care (Vaknin and Zisk-Rony 2011). Assent is described as non-refusal or simple agreement (Alderson 2007) with decisions made by others and as not requiring much knowledge and understanding (Hallström and Elander 2005). The elements of assent have been more recently described as information, comprehension, voluntariness and voluntary agreement (Ford 2010), which implies a greater level of understanding and not the simple agreement described in some work.

It is frequently the minor decisions of everyday care which are enforced on children without their views being heard (Coyne and Kirwan 2012; Hallström and Elander 2004; Livesley and Long 2013; Lowes 1996). Often there are missed opportunities for children and young people to become involved in choices and decisions and to provide their assent for nursing interventions. Everyday choices can include the location of where procedures take place and who is present. Simple measures including asking which arm children want their blood pressure taking on, or whether they would prefer tablet or liquid medicine. Opening up choices like these can provide children and young people with an opportunity to express an opinion and increase their co-operation. Health professionals have been shown to engage children in participating in the 'soft decisions' during hospitalisation, such as what to eat and drink and whether they want their parents close by, but involved them less in decisions about taking samples and examinations to be performed (Runeson et al. 2002). In some cases even the small choices such as food preferences and sleeping times are not given to children and young people and they have reported feeling as though they have to just fit in with a ward schedule (Coyne 2006b). There is less known about what involvement children and young people have in choices about aspects of their health care outside the acute care setting, such as when their care is carried out in schools, the community and within their own homes.

Some choices made by children and young people relate to who they share information with about their condition. In some cases these choices are not respected by professionals. The following excerpt illustrates how children's choices can be undermined by professionals. This 9-year-old boy managed information about his condition carefully, and only a few select friends both at school and within his social circle knew about his condition. It had been decided (between the teacher and the boy's parent) that prior to a school trip it would be better for classmates to understand his continence management regime to prevent awkward questions being asked. His mother described how

> '[the] *class were all sat down round a table and had a talk. They knew there was something wrong and they said 'when we go away* [child's name] *has got to go to the toilet and stay there for an hour, so any questions and you can ask him now, but after that, it is all forgot about'.* When the boy was asked how this decision had been made and how he felt about it, he was clear that it was 'the teacher' who made the decision and that he was 'not happy with the decision to tell everyone'. (Bray 2010:147)

Challenges can be encountered when children do not provide assent for a procedure which is deemed important or necessary by health professionals. If a child is seen to understand the reason for a procedure then his or her dissent ought to be taken seriously (Walker and Doyon 2001). This can be complex to apply in practice, for example, if a cannula is to be inserted or blood taken there are few young children who would sit still and offer their hand while this is carried out; they may get upset, wriggle and demonstrate their dissent for the procedure. This lack of co-operation with the cannulation can be seen as demonstrating a lack of the ability to weigh up short-term pain against long-term benefit (Hallström and Elander 2004). In order for a procedure to be carried out safely and quickly, children and young people may have to be held; this could be seen as going against their dissent. Runeson et al. (2001) provides a particularly upsetting example where a 9-year-old boy's protests at the removal of his stitches are ignored.

> As we try he kicks and hits furiously. Swears and screams, does not cry. We try to sedate him, but he refuses oral medicine and nasal spray. Finally the surgeon on call is brought in. He enters the room, and in a determined voice he tells the boy to lie down. The boy is held down while the stitches are removed. (Runeson et al. 2001: 73)

It is not clear in this scenario whether the boy's parents are present or to what extent the boy had been prepared for the procedure, but it is certain that he is not providing assent and has made the decision he does not want the procedure to go ahead at this time, in this way. Observed cases of clinical procedures have highlighted how the recommended practice of informing children and young people and providing them with opportunities to make choices can be overruled when parents and professionals prioritise getting a procedure done quickly over the expressed dissent of children and young people (Bray et al. 2012). Such situations are distressing for all, not least the child, and present a real concern for children's nurses faced with children who resist procedures. In contrast to those children who make their dissent known, either through physical or verbal means, it is the children who are quiet and shy who are the most likely to have their needs and voices overlooked (Livesley and Long 2013).

The findings of national UK inquiries into the medical treatment of children and young people have advised that consent should precede every clinical intervention and all 'touching' (Alderson 2007). This would cause health professionals potential problems in the case above or with any children who refuse to have minor proce-dures carried out and require holding.

Children and young people can express their assent and dissent in a variety of ways, such as through silence, cries, gestures and posture (Children's Hospitals Australasia 2010). Health care staff need to be aware and responsive to these cues. It is important to equally recognise the anxiety and dissent of a quiet, withdrawn child as much as a child who is actively crying and resisting. Recognising hidden or less visible communication signs can be difficult, but it is of particular impor-tance when working with children and young people with communication difficul-ties. Children who are ventilator dependent have reported that they were frequently excluded from decisions or unable to express their opinion about procedures due to a lack of availability of a suitable communication system (Noyes 2000). Com-munication with some children and young people needs dedicated staff and time, as well as ensuring that systems and relationships are established so that they can express an opinion. Although there is increasing recognition of the need to involve children and young people in decision making, implementation of this is slower

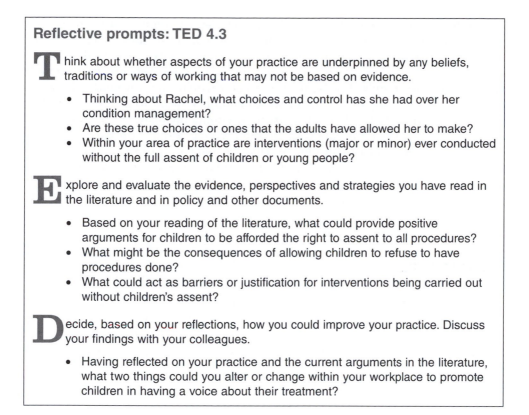

Reflective prompts: TED 4.3

Think about whether aspects of your practice are underpinned by any beliefs, traditions or ways of working that may not be based on evidence.

- Thinking about Rachel, what choices and control has she had over her condition management?
- Are these true choices or ones that the adults have allowed her to make?
- Within your area of practice are interventions (major or minor) ever conducted without the full assent of children or young people?

Explore and evaluate the evidence, perspectives and strategies you have read in the literature and in policy and other documents.

- Based on your reading of the literature, what could provide positive arguments for children to be afforded the right to assent to all procedures?
- What might be the consequences of allowing children to refuse to have procedures done?
- What could act as barriers or justification for interventions being carried out without children's assent?

Decide, based on your reflections, how you could improve your practice. Discuss your findings with your colleagues.

- Having reflected on your practice and the current arguments in the literature, what two things could you alter or change within your workplace to promote children in having a voice about their treatment?

with respect to children with disabilities (Franklin and Sloper 2009) compared to their peers who have no disabilities; this is especially so for children who need communication equipment.

The role of children's nurses

Throughout this chapter it is clear that involving children and young people in decisions and choices about their health care and management creates many opportunities and challenges. Health professionals have an important role in facilitating the involvement of children and young people in decisions about their health care and giving them the opportunity to become competent decision makers (Mårtenson and Fägerskiöld 2008; McPherson and Thorne 2000). Children's nurses have a key responsibility to build respectful and trusting relationships with children and young people so they feel able to report on their own lives. Although facilitating decision making is identified as an important and integral part of being a children's nurse, it is also seen by children's nurses as one of the most challenging aspects (Miller 2001). Nurses act as advocates for children and young people and, in turn, children see nurses as important to their decision-making process as they help interpret information from their parents and health professionals and help to structure the flow of information over time (Deatrick 1984).

Health professionals work in varied and complex situations and contexts, and many treatment decisions or choices are not made in a pre-organised, planned way. Involving children and young people in choices and decisions should be determined on an individual and situational basis and with discussion between professionals and a supportive family. Involvement and choices may focus around whether a medicine is given orally or rectally or who a child may want to be present while a cannula is inserted. These alternatives are more commonly ones which nursing staff will have to discuss and decide with children, young people and parents; nurses have an important role in advocating for children and young people and in facilitating how interventions and care are carried out (Hallström and Elander 2004). It is essential that nurses develop an understanding of the complex issues which are involved in promoting children and young people to be involved in health care choices and decisions.

Conclusion

Assessing the competence of children and young people to make decisions and choices can be complex, difficult, challenging and subjective. This should not prevent or dissuade professionals working with children and young people from spending time and providing opportunities for them to express their opinions, thoughts, concerns and preferences. Children and young people have better health care experiences when they have been given choices in how involved they are in decisions and they are generally competent to be involved in those choices and decisions if circumstances and influencing characteristics are taken into account. These characteristics include children's and young people's age, previous illness, health care and decision-making experience, the actions and inactions of health professionals, dynamics within the family, the context and environment they are in, their current health and the presence of illness symptoms. Health professionals are in a privileged position to be able to promote and support children and young people in making decisions and choices about their lives and health care; this will equip them for the decisions and choices which will be expected of them as they become young adults accessing adult health provision.

References

Alderson, P. (1993) *Children's Consent to Surgery*. Oxford: Open University Press.
Alderson, P. (2007) 'Competent children? Minors' consent to health care treatment and research', *Social Science & Medicine*, 65(11): 2272–2283.
Alderson, P. and Montgomery, J. (1996) *Health Care Choices: Making Decisions with Children*. London: Institute for Public Policy Research.
Angst, D.B. and Deatrick, J.A. (1996) 'Involvement in health care decisions: parents and children with chronic illness', *Journal of Family Nursing*, 2(2): 174–194.

Applebaum, P.S. (2007) 'Assessment of patients' competence to consent to treatment', *New England Journal of Medicine*, 357: 1834–40.

Atkin, K. and Ahmad, W. (2000) 'Living a normal life: young people with thalassaemia major or sickle cell disorder', *Social Science & Medicine*, 53(5): 615–626.

Baines, P. (2010) 'Death and best interests: a response to the legal challenge', *Clinical Ethics*, 5(4): 195–200.

Baines, P. (2011) 'Assent for children's participation in research is incoherent and wrong', *Archives of Disease in Childhood*, 96(10): 960–962.

Beauchamp, T.L. and Childress, J.F. (2001) *Principles of Biomedical Ethics*. New York: Oxford University Press, USA.

Beyth-Marom, R., Austin, L., Fischhoff, B., Palmgren, C. and Jacobs-Quadrel, M. (1993) 'Perceived consequences of risky behaviors: adults and adolescents', *Developmental Psychology*, 29(3): 549–563.

Billick, S.B., Edwards, J.L., Burgert, W. and Bruni, S. (1998) 'A clinical study of competency in child psychiatric inpatients', *Journal of the American Academy of Psychiatry and the Law Online*, 26(4): 587–594.

Boylan, P. (2004) *Children's Voices Project: Feedback From Children and Young People About Their Experience and Expectations of Healthcare*. Commission for Health Improvement.

Bray, L. (2007) 'Developing an activity to aid informed assent when interviewing children and young people', *Journal of Research in Nursing*, 12(5): 447–457.

Bray, L. (2010) 'Children, young people and their parents' experiences of having and living with a continent stoma'. Unpublished thesis, Manchester.

Bray, L., Callery, P. and Kirk, S. (2012) 'A qualitative study of the pre-operative preparation of children, young people and their parents for planned continence surgery: experiences and expectations', *Journal of Clinical Nursing*, 21(13–14): 1964–1973.

Bray, L., Kirk, S. and Callery, P. (2013) 'Developing biographies: the experiences of children, young people and their parents of living with a long-term condition', *Sociology of Health and Illness*, doi: 10.1111/1467-9566.12110.

Callery, P. and Milnes, L. (2012) 'Communication between nurses, children and their parents in asthma review consultations', *Journal of Clinical Nursing*, 21(11–12): 1641–1650.

Children's Hospitals Australasia (2010) *Charter on the Rights of Children and Young People in Healthcare Services in Australia*. Australia: Children's Hospitals Australasia.

Coad, J. and Houston, R. (2007) *Voices of Children and Young People. Involving Children and Young People in the Decision-making Processes of Healthcare Services. A Review of the Literature*. Report submitted to Action for Sick Children.

Coyne, I. (2006a) 'A review of children's decision-making competence in health care', *Journal of Clinical Nursing* 15(1): 61–71.

Coyne, I. (2006b) 'Children's experiences of hospitalization', *Journal of Child Health Care*, 10 (4): 326–36.

Coyne, I. (2006c) 'Consultation with children in hospital: children, parents' and nurses' perspectives', *Journal of Clinical Nursing*, 15(1): 61–71.

Coyne, I. and Harder, M. (2011) 'Children's participation in decision-making: balancing protection with shared decision-making using a situational perspective', *Journal of Child Health Care*, 15(4): 312–319.

Coyne, I. and Kirwan, L. (2012) 'Ascertaining children's wishes and feelings about hospital life', *Journal of Child Health Care*, 16(3): 293–304.

Crisp, J., Ungerer, J.A. and Goodnow, J.J. (1996) 'The impact of experience on children's understanding of illness', *Journal of Pediatric Psychology*, 21(1): 57–72.

Deatrick, J.A. (1984) 'It's their decision now: perspectives of chronically disabled adolescents concerning surgery', *Issues in Comprehensive Pediatric Nursing*, 7(1): 17–31.

Dovey-Pearce, G., Hurrell, R., May, C., Walker, C. and Doherty, Y. (2005) 'Young adults' (16–25 years) suggestions for providing developmentally appropriate diabetes services: a qualitative study', *Health & Social Care in the Community*, 13(5): 409–419.

Ellison, S. (2007) *The Best Interests of the Child in Healthcare*. London: Routledge and Cavendish.

Fiks, A.G., Hughes, C.C., Gafen, A., Guevara, J.P. and Barg, F.K. (2011) 'Contrasting parents' and pediatricians' perspectives on shared decision-making in ADHD', *Pediatrics*, 127(1): 188–196.

Ford, K. (2010) 'Reframing a sense of self: a constructivist grounded theory of children's admission to hospital for surgery'. Unpublished thesis, University of Tasmania.

Ford, K., Sankey, J. and Crisp, J. (2007) 'Development of children's assent documents using a child-centred approach', *Journal of Child Health Care*, 11(1): 19–28.

Franklin, A. and Sloper, P. (2009) 'Supporting the participation of disabled children and young people in decision-making', *Children & Society*, 23(1): 3–15.

Geist, R. and Opler, S.E. (2010) 'A guide for health care practitioners in the assessment of young people's capacity to consent to treatment', *Clinical Pediatrics*, 49(9): 834–839.

Hallström, I. and Elander, G. (2004) 'Decision-making during hospitalization: parents' and children's involvement', *Journal of Clinical Nursing*, 13(3): 367–375.

Hallström, I. and Elander, G. (2005) 'Decision making in paediatric care: an overview with reference to nursing care', *Nursing Ethics*, 12(3): 223–238.

Halpern-Felsher, B.L. and Cauffman, E. (2001) 'Costs and benefits of a decision: decision-making competence in adolescents and adults', *Journal of Applied Developmental Psychology*, 22(3): 257–273.

Hinds, P.S., Drew, D., Oakes, L., Fouladi, M, Spunt, S., Church, C. and Furman, W.L. (2005) 'End-of-life care preferences of pediatric patients with cancer', *Journal of Clinical Oncology*, 23(36): 9146–9154.

Hodges, F.M., Svoboda, J.S. and Van Howe, R.S. (2002) 'Prophylactic interventions on children: balancing human rights with public health', *Journal of Medical Ethics*, 28: 10–16

James, A. and Prout, A. (eds) (2004) *Constructing and Reconstructing Childhood: Contemporary Issues in the Sociological Study of Childhood*. London: Falmer Press.

Kilicarslan-Toruner, E. and Akgun-Citak, E. (2013) 'Information-seeking behaviours and decision-making process of parents of children with cancer', *European Journal of Oncology Nursing*, 17(2): 176–183.

Knopf, J.M., Hornung, R.W., Slap, G.B., DeVellis, R.F. and Britto, M.T. (2008) 'Views of treatment decision making from adolescents with chronic illnesses and their parents: a pilot study', *Health Expectations*, 11(4): 343–354.

Kunin, H. (1997) 'Ethical issues in pediatric life-threatening illness: dilemmas of consent, assent, and communication', *Ethics & Behavior*, 7(1): 43–57.

Lambert, V., Glacken, M. and McCarron, M. (2008) '"Visible-ness": the nature of communication for children admitted to a specialist children's hospital in the Republic of Ireland', *Journal of Clinical Nursing*, 17(23): 3092–3102.

Leikin, S. (1989) 'A proposal concerning decisions to forgo life-sustaining treatment for young people', *The Journal of Pediatrics*, 115(1): 17–22.

Leshin, L. (2000) 'Plastic surgery in children with Down syndrome', *Down Syndrome: Health Issues: News and Information for Parents and Professionals*, 30: 2008.

Levi, R.B., Marsick, R., Drotar, D. and Kodish, E.D. (2000) 'Diagnosis, disclosure, and informed consent: learning from parents of children with cancer', *Journal of Pediatric Hematology/Oncology*, 22(1): 3–12.

Levinson, W., Kao, A., Kuby, A. and Thisted, R.A. (2005) 'Not all patients want to participate in decision making', *Journal of General Internal Medicine*, 20(6): 531–535.

Lin, M., Pang, M.S. and Chen, C. (2013) 'Family as a whole: elective surgery patients' perception of the meaning of family involvement in decision making', *Journal of Clinical Nursing*, 22(1–2): 271–278.

Livesley, J. and Long, T. (2013) 'Children's experiences as hospital in-patients: voice, competence and work. Messages for nursing from a critical ethnographic study', *International Journal of Nursing Studies*, 50(10): 1292–1303.

Lowes, L. (1996) 'Paediatric nursing and children's autonomy', *Journal of Clinical Nursing*, 5(6): 367–372.

Mårtenson, E.K. and Fägerskiöld, A.M. (2008) 'A review of children's decision-making competence in health care', *Journal of Clinical Nursing*, 17(23): 3131–3141.

McAliley, L.G., Hudson-Barr, D.C., Gunning, R.S. and Rowbottom, L.A. (2000) 'The use of advance directives with adolescents', *Pediatric Nursing*, 26(5): 471–480.

McKenna, K., Collier, J., Hewitt, M. and Blake, H. (2010) 'Parental involvement in paediatric cancer treatment decisions', *European Journal of Cancer Care*, 19(5): 621–630.

McPherson, G. and Thorne, S. (2000) 'Children's voices: can we hear them?', *Journal of Pediatric Nursing*, 15(1): 22–29.

Meng, A. and McConnell, S. (2002) 'Decision-making in children with asthma and their parents', *Journal of the American Academy of Nurse Practitioners*, 14(8): 363–371.

Miller, S. (2001) 'Facilitating decision-making in young people', *Paediatric Nursing*, 13(5): 31–5.

Miller, V.A. (2009) 'Parent-child collaborative decision making for the management of chronic illness: a qualitative analysis', *Families, Systems & Health: The Journal of Collaborative Family Healthcare*, 27(3): 249–266.

National Health and Medical Research Council (2013) *National Statement on Ethical Conduct in Human Research*. Australian Government.

Noyes, J. (2000) 'Enabling young "ventilator-dependent" people to express their views and experiences of their care in hospital', *Journal of Advanced Nursing*, 31(5): 1206–15.

Noyes, J. (2007) 'Comparison of ventilator-dependent child reports of health-related quality of life with parent reports and normative populations', *Journal of Advanced Nursing*, 58(1): 1–10.

Pfeil, M. (2011) 'Parents' experience of giving consent for their child to undergo surgery', *Journal of Child Health Care*, 15(4): 380–388.

Piaget, J. (1924) *The Language and Thought of the Child*. London: Routledge.

Ross, L.F. (1998) *Children, Families, and Health Care Decision Making*. Oxford: Oxford University Press.

Royal College of Paediatrics and Child Health (RCPCH) (2000) 'Guidelines for the ethical conduct of medical research involving children', *Archives of Disease in Childhood*, 82: 117–182.

Runeson, I., Enskär, K., Elander, G. and Hermerén, G. (2001) 'Professionals' perceptions of children's participation in decision making in healthcare', *Journal of Clinical Nursing*, 10(1): 70–78.

Runeson, I., Hallström, I., Elander, G. and Hermerén, G. (2002) 'Children's participation in the decision-making process during hospitalization: an observational study', *Nursing Ethics*, 9(6): 583–598.

Rutishauser, C., Esslinger, A., Bond, L. and Sennhauser, F. (2003) 'Consultations with adolescents: the gap between their expectations and their experiences', *Acta Paediatrica*, 92(11): 1322–1326.

Sanders, C. and Bray, L. (2013) 'Examining professionals' and parents' views of using transanal irrigation with children: understanding their experiences to develop a shared health resource for education and practise', *Journal of Child Health Care*, e-publication ahead of print.

Sanders, C., Carter, B. and Goodacre, L. (2011) 'Searching for harmony: parents' narratives about their child's genital ambiguity and reconstructive genital surgeries in childhood', *Journal of Advanced Nursing*, 67(10): 2220–2230.

Sanders, C., Carter, B. and Goodacre, L. (2012) 'Parents need to protect: influences, risks and tensions for parents of prepubertal children born with ambiguous genitalia', *Journal of Clinical Nursing*, 21(21–22): 3315–23.

Tates, K. and Meeuwesen, L. (2001) 'Doctor–parent–child communication: a (re)view of the literature', *Social Science & Medicine*, 52(6): 839–851.

UN General Assembly (1989) *Convention on the Rights of the Child*. Geneva: United Nations.

Vaknin, O. and Zisk-Rony, R. (2011) 'Including children in medical decisions and treatments: perceptions and practices of healthcare providers', *Child: Care, Health & Development*, 37(4): 533–539.

Walker, N.E. and Doyon, T. (2001) 'Fairness and reasonableness of the child's decision: a proposed legal standard for children's participation in medical decision making', *Behavioral Sciences & the Law*, 19(5–6): 611–636.

Weithorn, L.A. and Campbell, S.B. (1982) 'The competency of children and adolescents to make informed treatment decisions', *Child Development*, 56(3): 1589–1598.

Wheeler, R. (2006) 'Gillick or Fraser? A plea for consistency over competence in children: Gillick and Fraser are not interchangeable', *British Medical Journal* 332(754): 5807.

Chapter 5

How Settings Shape Children's and Young People's Care

Key points

- Children and families are cared for in diverse settings and consideration of the impact, tensions and challenges of the context of care is an essential component of caring for children and families.
- The introduction of technology, health professionals and health services into private family spaces such as the home can be both enabling and disabling for families.
- Health care delivery to children and families within their homes, changes previously held understandings of space and place.
- Nurses play an important role in not only ensuring the spaces of care are safe and developmentally appropriate but also facilitating the functioning of the family and all its members.

Key theories and concepts explored in this chapter are space, place, technology and boundaries.

Case study 5.1: Sarah

Setting the scene

Sarah was 12 years old – in three months' time she would be 13! She lived at home with her parents and 9-year-old brother Frankie. Frankie was 'special'; he was born different, he had cerebral palsy. This meant that he could not walk and although he tried could not speak very well although she usually knew what he wanted. He had a wicked laugh! She loved Frankie and she loved making him laugh. Now that he went to the 'special school' it almost felt like they were a normal family except for Simon and the others! Simon was Frankie's caregiver and 'the others' were the carers who came when Simon was away. He came into their house every afternoon in time to meet the van that brought Frankie home from school. It was Simon's job to help her parents by looking after Frankie after school, feeding, and bathing, entertaining him and getting him ready for bed at night.

(Continued)

(Continued)

They hadn't always had Simon but now Dad was out of town for work during the week and Frankie was growing, Mum needed help. Since Frankie had grown, their house had changed as well. Every corner and passageway seemed to hold equipment for Frankie; wheelchairs, hoists, feeding pumps! They had an ugly ramp leading up to the front door and their bathroom didn't look like any of her friends' bathrooms. No room for nice towels and cosmetics just bath seats and the smelly creams and potions for Frankie. She hated the fact that when she got home it wasn't just Mum, her and Frankie. Although Mum was usually home when she got in from school it was hard to tell her things with Simon around. It was easier to go to her room – there was only normal girl stuff in there! Sometimes she went to her friends' homes after school but she didn't want anyone to come to her place. Simon and the others were nice, she guessed, they seemed to care about Frankie, but weekdays just weren't the same as the weekends. At the weekends it was just Mum, Dad, Frankie and her; then they were just a normal family.

Introduction

In recent decades there has been increasing diversity in relation to where and how health care is delivered to children and families. Increased family participation, advances in medical management and technology as well as improved understanding of the impact of the illness experience, hospitalisation and institutionalisation on children and families has led to a reconsideration of the spaces and places in which health care is delivered. Care delivery to children and families is no longer restricted to the hospital ward or clinic, but happens in the home, the community centre, school, hospice, day care centre, or via phone, email, audio conferencing or remote monitoring systems. The rapid development of web-based technology and social networks mean that the possibilities now seem endless. This chapter will consider the spaces and places in which care is delivered, and the possibilities and challenges such diverse settings may pose for children, their families, nursing and the delivery of health care services to children.

The places and spaces of care

The increasing importance of nurses understanding what is often referred to as the 'landscapes of care' is now well recognised (Andrews and Moon 2005). The term 'landscapes of care' has been used to describe the complex embodied spaces and places which emerge from and through the delivery of care. The concept of 'landscapes of care' may include institutions such as hospitals and schools, the family and home setting, community landscapes which may be public (e.g., playgrounds), voluntary (e.g., sports clubs, parent support groups) and private (e.g., day care) as well as the transition spaces in-between (e.g., the mobility taxi). To fully understand these landscapes, examination of the macro level, such as how care is organised and by whom at a national and international level, as well as the micro level, such as what is happening in specific spaces such as the home, a hospital ward or nursery, is required. 'Landscapes' include not only the physical elements such as the child's bed, ramp, hoist and the appearance of these objects, but also the spatial elements such as how the space is perceived and interacted with in an emotional sense by the child and family. The temporal element relates to how these perceptions and responses change over time. Landscapes of care are not only the varied and often increasingly complex environments in which care is delivered but also the embodied nature of space and place and the interplay between the structures, processes and experiences of care (Milligan 2003). In the following section we will consider some of the most frequent 'landscapes of care' for children and young people with health care needs.

At home

One of the most frequent spaces in which care is delivered to children is within their own home. Increased understanding of the impact of hospitalisation and institution-alisation on children and families, the medical risks (e.g., cross infection, exposure to medical error) and psychosocial risks associated with hospitalisation (Board and Ryan-Wenger 2002; Caldas et al. 2004; Carnevale et al. 2006; Coyne 2006; Kearns and Collins 2000) and recognition of the expertise and competence of families to manage treatment and care in the home, has led to the home now being the preferred location for the delivery of health care to children (Vickers et al. 2007; Young et al. 2006). While in the past children would have only been considered as being safely and adequately cared for by health professionals within the confines of a hospital or long-term care facility, improvements in portable technology and home care support, as well as the expertise and increasing competence of families to manage their child's condition, have meant that children are more often cared for at home. For most children requiring long-term health care, hospital stays have become shorter and less frequent.

When considering the home as a place for health care delivery, nurses must examine this from a perspective that is wider than just a physical location or the space in which the family resides. The home is primarily a *place of meaning*. It is a place of connection and memories. A place which both develops and reinforces identity, sense of self and connection to others and the wider world. It is the place where values and roles are established, maintained and developed to enable family functioning and support those residing in it (Milligan 2003). For many it is seen as a private sanctuary, a place of comfort and security; a place to be a family. Caring for the child in the home offers the child and family the security and comfort of developing and maintaining vital family connections, allowing the family to create their own unique way of being. The introduction of health care into the home impacts not only on the family's view and understanding of home and the way in which their family functions and operates but also that embodied sense of being at home.

The majority of health care delivered in the home is delivered by the family themselves; however, most families will require intermittent visits from health professionals. Frequent visits and movement of health professionals and other care supporters in and out of the home and the introduction of equipment and technology brings with it challenges not only in regard to how the family functions but also to the experience and meaning of home.

Case study 5.2: Sarah

Being at home

Sarah's reference to 'the ramp' (physical structure and location), the space which Frankie's equipment occupies (spatial component), and the routines and timing of family activities (temporal), reflect this wider concept of being at home. Sarah describes it as a place where sometimes – at the weekend – they can 'just be a family'. A place where they can do what they like doing when they like doing it, where they invite or exclude membership, laugh, argue, debate, discipline, negotiate, celebrate and love privately, away from the scrutiny and view of others. That is why weekends are so special; they are 'at home' as a real family.

In the community

Another place where health care is often delivered to children is within community settings. These sites can be informal ones such as the shopping mall, the car, the playground or sports field, or formal settings such as community clinics, schools or day care centres. Caring for children in community settings allows the child/family to maintain social connectedness and the ability to participate in social, sport and community activities (Carnevale et al. 2006; Earle et al. 2006; Heaton et al. 2005; McKeever et al. 2002). However, the delivery of health care in community settings requires consideration of the environment the child is entering (e.g., accessibility, transport), exposure to risk (e.g., infection, injury), portability and the ability to transport and use treatments and equipment (e.g., power, medication storage) and the expertise and skills of community caregivers. Unlike the delivery of care in the home setting which can be carried out within the comfort, security, privacy and protection of the family home where the family has control of how and who delivers care to the child, caring in the community exposes the child and family not only to the gaze (judgement) of others but also to the prospect of perhaps handing care over to someone else. There is evidence which shows that being able to regularly participate in the wider community reduces children's isolation, improves their social skills, physical well-being and their ability to become part of society (Heaton et al. 2005; Hinckson et al. 2013; Imms et al. 2009; Yantzi et al. 2007); it also comes with challenges and tensions in relation to acceptance and safety. Despite many societies making considerable efforts to ensure inclusion, acceptance and participation of children with disability and illness in the community, research continues to show that families encounter prejudice, stigma and reactions from people which often make it difficult for them to feel part of the community to which they belong (Carnevale et al. 2006; Carter et al. 2014).

In the hospital

The hospital, while often now viewed as the least desirable place to deliver health care to children, from a psychosocial perspective is often a necessary location for care when the child's condition is such that they cannot be safely or adequately cared for at home or in the community. Growing awareness of the impact of hospitalisation on children has led to shorter hospital stays and the transformation of many hospitals into more child-friendly spaces. There is rising interest and research in the design of hospital buildings, with a trend to have the architecture not only more child friendly but also more reflective of places in the community which may have a more positive associations for children such as shopping malls, parks and playgrounds (Adams et al. 2010; Andrews 2004; Kearns and Barnett 2000). The Hospital in the Park, in Alder Hey, Liverpool, UK, which is due to be completed in Autumn 2015 has been designed with children's and young people's input; the curves, materials and design aim to create a child-friendly environment and it is positioned within a park that will be used by the community (see Figure 5.1).

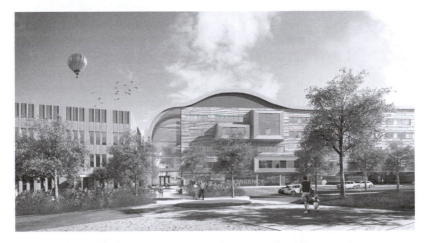

Figure 5.1   Architectural sketch of the Hospital in the Park, Alder Hey Children's NHSFT (used with kind permission of Alder Hey NSHFT)

For many families, frequent admissions may have led them to consider the hospital as a familiar space, a necessary sanctuary or even an extension of home. However, for many children and their families the hospital environment remains frightening and unfamiliar. Research has shown that despite the best attempts of architects, service providers and health professionals to make hospitals more child/family-friendly spaces, hospitalisation is still associated with negative psychosocial sequelae (anxiety, developmental and behavioural changes, post-traumatic stress disorder), separation and social disconnection, loss of power and control along with significant disruption to family life (Carney et al. 2003; Ford 2011).

In residential care or a long-term care facility

The use of 'out of home' residential care for children has significantly reduced in developed countries with the increase of home and community supports for children

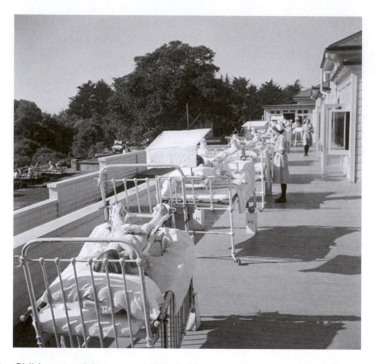

Figure 5.2   Children receiving care at Wilson Home, a long term care facility in Auckland,
New Zealand (circa 1943)

requiring long-term health care. Institutional care as reflected in the photo of children
being cared for in Aukland, New Zealand in 1943 is now rarely seen in developed
countries (see Figure 5.2). However, in some areas of the world, in particular Eastern
Europe, Central and South America, Africa and the Middle East, institutional care of
children is still seen as preferable and quite commonly used (Dozier et al. 2012). Even
in developed countries such Australia and the USA up to one-third of families caring
for children with severe disability may seek long-term or short-term placement for
their child outside of the family home (McConkey et al. 2004). There is an extensive
body of research which shows the detrimental effects of long-term institutional care
on children, including impairment in social and interpersonal development, physical
growth retardation, and delayed cognitive and language development (Dozier et al.
2012; Johnson et al. 2006). Many of these detrimental effects relate to the characteristics of many long-term residential care facilities: high child to staff ratios, untrained
caregivers, shift working, routine or regimented care and a lack of individualised
psychological care. However, even in well-run, well-staffed and well-resourced facilities, while less marked, the effects of institutionalisation are still seen (Dozier et al.
2012; Johnson et al. 2006). Despite the evidence which shows the detrimental effects
of residential care, many families still require and seek out 'out of home' care for their
children. The reasons given by families for doing so relate to the lack of local community-based supports and respite services, the families' inability to manage the care and

behaviours of the child especially as they get older, and the needs of other family members (Dozier et al. 2012; McConkey et al. 2004; Mirfin-Veitch et al. 2003; Sellick 1998). However, as Mirfin-Veitch et al. (2003) demonstrated, making this decision is not an easy one for families and it is generally a 'process rather than a discrete act' (p.109) as they carefully weigh up the options.

Case study 5.3: Sarah

Out of home care

Although Frankie has 'in-home respite care' and supports from a number of agencies, the family has begun to utilise residential 'out of home' respite care to allow the family to take a break from the demands of his care and for her parents to spend more time with Sarah. Like many families living in countries whose community-based support services have not kept pace with the closing of residential care (deinstitutionalisation), Frankie's parents worry what the future may hold for Frankie when they are no longer able to be the main care providers.

Remote care: telemedicine and beyond

With reduction in costs, development of information technologies (IT) and the availability and accessibility of wireless facilities, we have seen the increasing development of telemedicine and remote technologies. Many children and families can access information about their condition, search out options for management, conduct consultations or conversations with health professionals about their health and its management, and form their own support communities via a wide range of information and digital technologies (Bacigalupe 2011). We also now have the ability to monitor health and keep families connected with each other, even when the family is separated by distance or hospitalisation (Gray et al. 2000; Smith 2007). While the participation of children and families in this environment may involve expensive videoconferencing at a local clinic, the rapid development of the worldwide web (www) and social networking services such as Skype, Ustream, Twitter and Facebook have enabled increasing participation by children and families who have access to the internet. Use of such technologies gives families access to information more readily, overcomes time and distance barriers, and fosters resiliency; it also empowers families, enables decision-making and improves satisfaction with health services (Bacigalupe 2011; Gray et al. 2000; Hall and Irvine 2009; Smith 2007). Initial reluctance by some health professionals to consider or engage in this way with children and families due to concerns regarding privacy, security, boundary issues, and accessibility is gradually dissipating. It is now acknowledged that many of these concerns are just as evident in traditional 'face-to-face' communication, and the issues associated with use of IT are more about the health professionals' understanding of the technologies and their ability to adapt to the different speed and medium of communication. Smith-Stoner (2011) demonstrated that with clearly established procedural, behavioural and privacy standards,

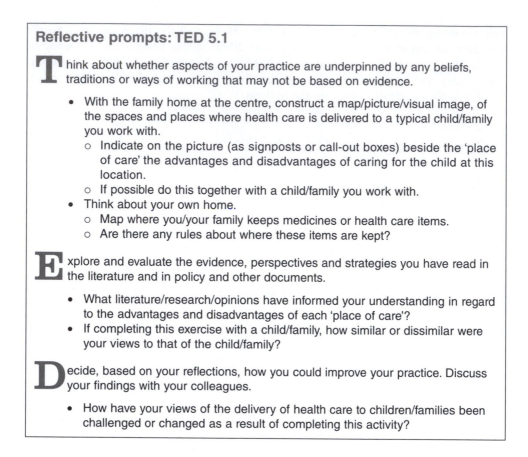

families can be safely supported in the community using IT. Bacigalupe (2011) describes how, for clinicians such as nurses, it is not *will* we engage in this virtual world but *how* we will engage.

The spaces and places of health care delivery have expanded rapidly in the last decade. There is evidence that, in most instances, the expansion of care sites mitigates many of the negative aspects of the illness experience for children and families. However, there are also challenges and tensions for children, families and nurses. Changes in the spaces and places of care impact not only on families but also on nurses, other health professionals and carers, who need to reconsider and adapt the way in which they work with families across diverse settings and mediums.

The impact of health care on child and family space

In the previous section we examined and explored the diverse environments in which health care can be delivered to children. The introduction and delivery of health care in such diverse settings often requires the introduction of technology, health professionals, caregivers, health services and organisations into spaces and places not intended for health care delivery. This can be enabling, reunifying the family and supporting family functioning and care of the child in a safe, secure, familiar and comfortable setting. Health care, however, may impact on the physical structures and appearance of the home, and the routines, roles and responsibilities of the child and family (Kirk 2010; Vickers and Carlisle 2000; Young et al. 2006). Delivery of care in diverse settings brings tensions and challenges not only for the child and family but also for nurses caring for families. This section will consider the impact of technology, health professionals, other services and caregivers on children and families receiving health care and encourage consideration of ways in which nurses might mitigate any adverse effects.

Technology in the home

The intrusion of equipment and technology into the family space may be on a large scale, for example a home ventilator or dialysis machine; however, frequently the impact is small and easily hidden from public view, such as occurs with a spacer device, a walker, or a medication fridge. While the impact of the technology on the home may be minimal as it becomes incorporated into the fabric of the home and family life, the technologies remain markers of difference for that family.

There is a growing body of research which looks at the impact of placing medical equipment and technology into the home setting. Many studies have been set in the context of children requiring complex technologies such as home ventilation (Carnevale et al. 2006; Darvill et al. 2009; Earle et al. 2006), but there has also been some consideration of technology which would now be considered less complex, such as feeding pumps, suction machines and tracheostomies (Heaton et al. 2005; Kirk 2010; Moore et al. 2010). Family and child perspectives have been evaluated – however, most studies have looked specifically at technology in the home setting, with only marginal reference to the impact of using medical devices in wider community settings.

It has been suggested that the introduction of technology is often viewed more positively by the children than their parents (Darvill et al. 2009), and that for many children who have used medical devices for some time the technology often becomes a physical extension of their body (Kirk 2010). Children have often been positive about the inclusion of medical devices in their care, noting that it has been helpful in assisting with their functional limitations, fostering their independence and ability to do, as Darvill et al. (2009) explained, the 'normal things'. The introduction of medical technology has been noted to improve physical health and energy, reduce hospital admissions and enable greater understanding of the child and their family in regard to their illness, medical care and treatments (Earle et al. 2006; Heaton et al. 2005; Huang et al. 2009; Kirk 2010). However, there is evidence to suggest that this positive view of technology may be context- and purpose-specific. Huang et al. (2009) demonstrated that children with cerebral palsy are more comfortable using assistive devices at school where it enhances school performance and their ability to engage with peers compared to its use in the more relaxed and leisurely environment of the home. In contrast, Earle et al. (2006) and Heaton et al. (2005) in their studies of children on assisted ventilation demonstrated that children showed a preference to keep the technology in the private sphere of the home because it was deemed to be difficult to integrate into the school routine and environment, required explanation and interfered with peer relationships. All the evidence suggests that medical technology does intrude on the child's sense of place and space, impacting not only on their physical disturbance and comfort but also on how they are perceived by others and interact with the world. There is also growing evidence to suggest that children, particularly older children and young people, are uncomfortable with the medicalisation of their personal spaces such as bedrooms and with the increased surveillance by a wider group of adults of their actions and behaviours (Kholen et al. 2000; Kirk 2010). Moore and Carter (2012: 13) discuss the notion of 'persistent ambivalence' to describe how recipients of home-based assistive technologies are both 'simultaneously grateful and resentful'.

Families, therefore, can be both enabled and disabled by the introduction of technology into their lives. Technology is enabling for families by reducing hospitalisation and disturbance to family functioning and by improving family understanding, confidence and competence in relation to the child's disability and illness. However, it has also been shown to be disabling by isolating or impeding families' connections with their usual social networks and increasing demands on parental time and family finance (Carnevale et al. 2006).

The introduction of technology into the home may require changes to the physical structure of the home to accommodate and support equipment and medical devices. Often families are able to preserve the comfort of the family space by disguising or concealing the technology, but often it remains as visible markers of difference for the child and family. As equipment is introduced, private, public and personal spaces within the home may change, impacting not only on the child but also on individual family members.

Case study 5.4: Sarah

Markers of difference

For Sarah the ramp, wheelchair, hoist, feeding pump and creams and potions in the bathroom are all visible markers that this is not a normal family space. From Sarah's perspective Frankie's occupation of the home appears to be expanding; there are few places within the home now which don't contain some of Frankie's things. Sarah feels that her only space of comfort within the home now is her bedroom.

The introduction of technology usually demands changes to family routines and responsibilities, sometimes reducing the time the parents have to spend with other children and family members or participate in sport and social functions. Assistive technology used to support children with long-term illness/disability can both enable independence and demand dependence. Assistive technology can increase the burden of care or reduce it. No matter how simple or complex, medical technology and equipment does change the meaning and functioning of the spaces and places children and families occupy (Moore and Carter 2012). Children and families will respond differently so it is important that this impact is acknowledged and considered whenever assistive technology is introduced into the care of the child.

Health professionals and carers

The places and spaces of care also impact on how families and nurses work together. As families and nurses move between health care settings, changes occur in relationship to proximity, roles and responsibilities and power and authority, and nurses and families are challenged to constantly adapt and renegotiate relationships to account for different settings and ways of engaging.

When a child and family enters a health care service they find themselves, perhaps for the first time ever, in proximity to nurses and other health professionals. However, in whatever setting, home or hospital, it is not just the objective measure of physical distance between nurse and family which determines proximity but how the nurse and family interact with each other. Malone (2003) describes three interrelated modes of proximity which may be evident in nursing: physical proximity, where the nurse engages in the physical act of touching and caring for the child/family; narrative proximity, where the nurse takes the opportunity to hear and understand the family story; and moral proximity, where through proximity the nurse recognises the need to be with or act for the child/family. Using Malone's approach it is possible to see that it is not just geographical distance – whether the care is delivered in the hospital or home – which creates the sense of proximity, but how the nurse, child and family engage with each other.

Case study 5.5: Sarah

Proximity

Although Frankie's father may be geographically and physically disconnected from the family during the week he remains proximal in the narrative and moral sense to Frankie's care through his nightly 'check-in' phone calls to the family. Equally, Simon (the carer) may be physically proximal to Frankie in that he engages in physical caring for much of the day; however, his time with Frankie is limited and often the family are not present so he has had limited opportunities to hear the family's stories (narratives) which would enable a genuine understanding of the family's perspective. This and his scope of practice does not allow him the moral proximity described by Malone (2003). Simon's proximity to Frankie often acts as a barrier to Sarah connecting with Frankie and her parents. For Frankie's parents, Simon's proximity to Frankie provides the reassurance they need that Frankie would remain safe and well.

Ideally, nurses will encounter all aspects of proximity in their practice with the child and family, but some authors argue that the reorganisation of health care delivery and the increasing use of carers to provide care to children is distancing nurses from the families they care for and that this is as prevalent in the hospital as the home setting (Bender et al. 2009; Malone 2003; Peter and Liaschenko 2004). While Malone (2003) urges nurses to remain proximal to their patients regardless of the geographical setting in which they work, there is a growing body of nursing literature which highlights the potential moral distress which can occur if the nurses are not adequately resourced and supported. Proximity, therefore, is as much a subjective experience as a geographical one and will often be perceived differently by the child, individual family members and nurses.

As discussed earlier, the different spaces and places in which health care is delivered influence the roles and responsibilities of nurses and families, and with this comes the challenging issue of power and control which will impact on how the nurse and family work together. In the health care facility, the responsibility for care and treatment, while to some extent shared, is usually legally mandated as the responsibility of the health professional and health care organisation. However, when care is delivered in the home the roles and responsibilities are less obvious. In this space there is more potential for role conflict and a need for clear negotiation and agreement on roles and responsibilities (Milligan 2003; Poland et al. 2005; Young et al. 2006). The difference in the nature of the relationship between nurse and family in the hospital and home has often somewhat simplistically been described as nurse as host (in the hospital setting) and nurse as guest (in the community setting), with authority and power resting with the family in the home and the nurse in the hospital. However, there is a growing awareness that this is a rather simplistic view and that regardless of the setting, power and authority may and indeed should ebb and flow between family and nurse (Bender et al. 2009; Dickinson et al. 2006; Wilson 2001). Unfortunately, nurses can fail to recognise this changing power dynamic and this may lead to tensions in regard to how care is both delivered and received (Milligan 2003; Poland et al. 2005).

Related to the notion of power and authority is the concept of surveillance. The very nature of nursing work, even in the primary health care setting, is often associated with surveillance of child and family. Surveillance may be in relation to whether treatment is being followed, responses to treatment or monitoring of growth development, all of which are aspects of nursing which nurses caring for children and young people regularly engage in. Health care spaces within hospitals and the technology used within the home are often designed specifically to facilitate surveillance, and, as discussed earlier in the chapter, the introduction of information technologies opens up new possibilities for surveillance by nurses in the home and community. This influences how nurses and families perceive and interact with each other in these places. A number of studies of families' experience of health care have noted the tension and challenge that the watchful gaze of the nurses can exert on families both in hospital and community settings (Carnevale et al. 2006; Kirk 2010; McKeever et al. 2002). The appearance of the space they occupy, be it the home or hospital room, is often perceived by families, and unfortunately sometimes nurses, as an indicator of their ability to competently care for and manage the child's health care needs. Families often prioritise tidying and cleaning their home prior to the nurse's visit to ensure that the appearance of their child and home means that they are judged as a competent carer for the child. Equally, as Bender describes, nurses working in the community may buy into value laden geographical labels such as a 'poor area', 'low socioeconomic area', 'a housing estate' or 'affluent area' and make stereotypical judgements based on where in the town/city/village the family live (Bender et al. 2009). As the spaces and places of care become more diverse it will be necessary for nurses to consider the impact the context of care has on their relationships with families and develop new and innovative ways of working with families.

This section has reviewed the impact of health care being delivered in diverse settings, many of which are not specifically designed or intended for health care delivery. The introduction of health care into such diverse settings blurs the boundaries between private and public space and challenges and changes the meaning of the space for child and family, especially when technology is introduced. As children and families move between locations they must constantly renegotiate roles, responsibilities and boundaries with health professionals and other carers. Nurses need to consider the impact of

---

Reflective prompts: TED 5.2

Think about whether aspects of your practice are underpinned by any beliefs, traditions or ways of working that may not be based on evidence.

- Consider the situation of a child/family you are currently caring for/or would usually care for in your practice.
- Make a list of all the services and equipment you believe will be required to care for this child/family.
- Try and imagine how much space it takes up and where you would place and/or store it in your own home.
  - How would it make you feel if you had to accommodate some of these items within your own home?
  - Why would you have these feelings?

Explore and evaluate the evidence, perspectives and strategies you have read in the literature and in policy and other documents.

- Review the list and identify what literature, research, policy, clinical guidelines and expert opinion supports each item on your list.
- How might each item enable or disable the child and family?
- What are the key issues which need to be taken into account in relation to ensuring the safety of the child and their family in relation to these items?
- What do the local policies state about professional boundaries when caring for a child in their own home?

Decide, based on your reflections, how you could improve your practice. Discuss your findings with your colleagues.

- Reflecting on this activity and what you have read, what recommendations would you make to enhance the enabling factors?
- What measures might you and the family explore to help reduce the impact of the disabling factors?

their presence and the services they deliver on the family, cognisant that this may vary between family members. They must also be willing to be flexible and adaptable in relation to how and where services are delivered and engage families in decision making, not only about what services will be delivered but where and how they will be delivered.

Maintaining spaces and places for children and their families

The complexity and challenges of delivering health care to children in increasingly diverse settings calls on nurses to consider innovative and flexible ways of providing care. They need to enable and maintain the family space and functioning but also ensure that the child and family receive the health services and care they require. Strategies which may need to be considered will vary considerably based on the child's illness, the cultural context in which care is delivered, the resources and services available, geographical proximity or distance from health services and, most importantly, the values, goals and aspirations of the family. For the family with a child with a long-term illness or disability the interplay between these factors will be dynamic as the child and family develop and circumstances and services change. Rather than providing a comprehensive list of strategies for 'how to' address these issues, this section will propose some underlying principles which could be used when planning and delivering health services to children and families.

Enabling and maintaining family space

As discussed earlier in this chapter, the introduction of health services into previously private spaces such as the family home changes the nature and functioning of the family and their home. Challenges also arise when attempting to create 'home like' age-appropriate spaces in public institutions such as hospitals and respite care facilities. Some attention has been given to the design and architecture of children's and young people's health care services so that they are 'home like' and meet the needs of children, young people and their families (Adams et al. 2010; Andrews 2004; Hutton 2005; Kearns and Barnett 2000). However, other than noting the importance of considering children and their family, the acceptability and impact of the environment and issues of privacy, little attention has been paid to how family space is negotiated or maintained in either the home or the hospital/institutional setting. Studies have been undertaken in older adult long-term facilities where staff have set out to constitute the hospital as home by making the environment and relationship with staff more 'home like'. However, as Gilmour (2006) describes, this is by no means straightforward and does not necessarily overcome the tensions already discussed in relation to roles, boundaries and vulnerability. Gilmour (2006), in reviewing the older adult setting, suggests that perhaps rather than a focus on creating a home in the institutional or hospital setting, which can be problematic, the focus wherever nursing care is delivered should be on creating an environment which privileges the nurse–patient relationship and maintains identity and personal expression. Gilmour's suggestion provides a sound basis for the nursing of children and young people, with the addition of environments which are cognisant and enabling of the developmental needs of children and their families.

Three principles for enabling and maintaining family space in the context of health care delivery to children and families need to be considered.

1. Recognition and affirmation of how the delivery of health care impacts on the child, individual family members, family functioning and previously held understandings of home and privacy.
2. Negotiation and agreement on private and shared spaces for the child, family, individual family members, nurses and other health care workers.
3. Established mechanisms for how boundaries will be maintained, renegotiated and traversed when delivering health care to the child.

Affirming the impact

As discussed previously, the movement of child and family into a health care setting and health care into the home or community, changes not only how the child and family function but also previously held understandings of being 'at home'. Familiar spaces become unfamiliar and unfamiliar spaces may become an extension of home. Nurses and the family must acknowledge that, for a while at least, feelings of 'at homeness' will be challenged (Moore and Carter 2012). Nurses and families need to take time to establish what is important in relation to maintaining family function. They need to understand the impact of treatments and technology, how, when and where health services are delivered, and the needs and aspirations of the child, individual family members and the family as a whole. It is important to affirm that no matter what attempts are made to minimise the impact of treatments and services the nature and meaning of spaces and places will change.

Case study 5.6: Sarah

Changes to our home

Sarah's relationship not only with her family and how she has come to understand and operate in her home has changed as a result of changes in Frankie's care. While Sarah's parents have been involved in numerous 'case meetings' where decisions have been made regarding what services will be delivered, what equipment is to be introduced and physical structures which would need to change in the home, Sarah has until now been excluded from this decision-making process. The focus of the case meetings with the

(Continued)

(Continued)

parents has been all about Frankie, with little consideration of the impact this may have on Sarah as she moves into her adolescent years. The increased presence of 'Frankie's stuff' in the home was unanticipated and the introduction of a wider range of services into Frankie's care has brought with it compromises in relation to how the family functions. It was not until Sarah's recent 'outburst', as her parents call it, that they became aware of how much the nature of their home had changed and how much they had accommodated family life to care for Frankie. How different might Sarah's story have been if the nurses and other health professionals had sat down with the whole family at each decision point and discussed what was important to them as a family, the impact that care decisions may have on those things and the potential alternatives available to them. Simple actions can be effective, like allowing family to view and try equipment and services prior to introducing them into the home. How different may Sarah's story have been if her parents and health professionals had asked her what was important to her in regard to home and family life and included her in some of the decision making, providing her with some options of how her needs might also be accommodated along the way?

Nurses must also consider how children and families may come to hospitals and services. For some these are familiar places to visit; acknowledgement of past experiences and connections to the environment are important, as is recognition that their individual needs and preferences are noted and remembered. For these families their need is to be re-orientated to the ward or service rather than being treated as a newcomer. For another family the hospital space may be quite alien, the bed and bedroom look nothing like that of home, despite the colourful pictures on the wall and teddy bear curtains. This family will come with some understandings of what hospital is like from stories, television or past family experiences but until now they have not experienced living in hospital as a family. The family may never have experienced living communally in a room with four other families separated only by a flimsy curtain. Unsure of the location of the bathroom or kitchen, even the basic tasks which they can usually perform for each other with ease (e.g. preparing and eating food, bathing and play) become difficult. The sights, sounds and smells of this space can be both unfamiliar and frightening. The hospital or clinic may have attempted to make this place 'like home' but it is not home. This family will require a very different approach with regard to the space they now occupy. For this family, the nurse must take time to familiarise them with the hospital, the location of services, and the sights and sounds they may hear. It will be important for the nurse to ascertain the things that may make them more comfortable in this space and where possible accommodate these, such as a special pillow, music player, family photos. A hospital space is not likely to be like home but the nurse can create features that are 'home like' and which can perhaps provide an anchor point for child and family. Whatever strategies the nurse or family utilise to create family space, both must come to understand that the nature and meaning of the space the family now occupy will have changed and that there will be periods of discomfort as the family and health service change and adapt to accommodate the delivery of health care to the child.

Defining the spaces

There have been a number of studies which have examined the experience of children and families living in hospitals (Ford 2011; Hopia et al. 2005; McKeever et al. 2002) and having health care delivered in the home (Carnevale et al. 2006; Carter et al. 2012; Darvill et al. 2009; Heaton et al. 2005; Vickers and Carlisle 2000). A common theme in many of these studies is the issue of self-determination and the tensions of establishing and maintaining private family space. Nurses need to negotiate and define the spaces of care, whether care is being delivered in the home or hospital setting. Shared spaces include places where family and health providers may work together, treatment spaces designated for administering treatments to the child, and social spaces reserved for family play, entertainment and socialising. Private spaces include those reserved for individual family members or just for the family. The boundaries of shared and private spaces need to be established. These will not necessarily be set geographical locations, particularly in the home setting, but the health provider and family should work together to determine how these spaces will be defined and renegotiated.

In the hospital setting such locations may already be determined through allocated rooms such as the treatment room, play room, bed space, parents' lounge, nurses' station, staff room, etc. However, even within these settings, studies have shown that the boundaries are not always maintained or clearly defined, often causing conflict and tension between children, families and health providers (Arlidge et al. 2009; Avis and Reardon 2008; Espezel 2003). The reality is that even within hospitals and clinics, boundaries often need to move based on the needs of the child, the availability of equipment, staff and resources, and the changes in treatment approaches. Nurses cannot assume that spaces are defined by signs and hospital regulations, as even the language used on signs may be unfamiliar to the family. Nurses need to engage the child and family in coming to understand the location they find themselves in and work with them to define shared and private spaces for both family and staff during the duration of the hospital stay.

Within the home, determining shared and private spaces becomes more complex, with the boundaries perhaps having to be flexible depending on the time of day, day of the week, the occupants and the activities occurring. As with any home there will be conflicts and compromise, but nurses delivering care in the home must remain aware that just as the family is not free to roam and occupy every part of a hospital facility so too they cannot assume that they have free range of the home. Care must be delivered in such a way that the shared and private spaces of the family are respected, maintained and encouraged.

Case study 5.7: Sarah

Changing private family and treatment spaces

For Sarah, private and family spaces contract during the week when Simon (the carer) is present and expand during the weekend when only family members are present in the house. The presence of Frankie's equipment and 'potions' in almost every room in the house

(Continued)

> *(Continued)*
>
> now suggest that all these spaces operate as both shared family space and treatment space for Frankie. Perhaps Sarah may view her home differently if it were possible for Frankie's equipment to be stored in just one or two locations in the house and/or disguised or put away in a cupboard when not in use. This would make it less visible in the shared spaces in the home. If Sarah was given the opportunity to participate in redesigning how the bathroom space is used so it can accommodate her special toiletries and make-up as well as Frankie's needs, this might make her feel more comfortable using the bathroom. It could be relatively simple to organise Frankie's care in such a way that after school there is a designated space in the house where Simon will not enter so that she can sit and chat uninterrupted with her mother.

Negotiating and maintaining the boundaries

One of the most difficult areas which challenge both families and nurses is how private and shared spaces are negotiated and maintained within both hospital and home settings. Frequently tensions arise in relation to how the boundaries around child, family and treatment have been negotiated and maintained. Nurse, child and family can never assume that the boundaries are clear and that they can and will remain the same for that child and family over time. Unfortunately, assumptions are often made and frank and open discussions about the reasons for the boundaries between spaces, the need for them to change and the rules around how boundaries are maintained, traversed and negotiated are not openly discussed. The spaces of care will change frequently and for differing reasons, what is important is that these are openly negotiated and explained. As with defining spaces, there will often be a need for compromise related to the needs of the child and, in some instances, legal, ethical and safety issues, not only for the child and family but also for those caring for the child.

> ## Case study 5.8: Sarah
>
> ### Shifting boundaries
>
> Sarah appears to have established a clear boundary in relation to who may enter her bedroom but she no longer seems to feel comfortable traversing other shared spaces in the home when Simon is present. Equally, her comfort about bringing her friends into the family home seems to have diminished. This is now a difficult place for her to bring her friends into and she now frequently socialises outside of the home. While in many ways this may reflect her transition into adolescence, it is also an indicator that, for the moment at least, the private, shared and treatment spaces in her home have not been clearly defined or negotiated. Similarly, the family have discovered that even in the clinic and hospital the boundaries often change, reflecting the differing attitudes of staff. While on some visits it is OK for Frankie to be left behind the nurses' station while the family go for some tea, at

other times the 'staff only' rule for this area is strictly enforced. While sometimes it is OK for Sarah stay alone and entertain Frankie for short periods while her Mum collects some laundry (as she would at home), at other times her mother is challenged for leaving her alone in the ward with Frankie.

Legal and regulatory influences

In addition to defining the spaces and places for care and how they will be traversed, it is important to consider the local legal and regulatory requirements which might influence where and how a child is cared for. These may relate to the physical, psychological, cultural and developmental safety of the child, family and carer. For example, the provision of an approved hoist, feeding pumps and ramps has to meet requirements for building regulations and safety. Requirements and regulations are different in different settings and apply to health and educational standards. Charters and cultural safety regulations may determine who may care for the child and in what circumstances. Regulations may also set out the cultural, developmental and educational supports and services to which the child (and family) must have access to ensure the psychological well-being of the child. These requirements will vary between countries and, in some instances, between regions within a country. Nurses must be aware of the cultural and regulatory requirements in their area which may influence how the child and family are cared for, ensuring that the family receive appropriate advice and assistance. Often there will be challenges in relation to what services are involved and where care is delivered and by whom. Other challenges include upholding the rights of the child and their family to self-determination versus the government's role in ensuring the protection and safety of the child. This can become a delicate balancing act between comfort and safety.

In addition to physical and psychological safety when delivering health care to children, consideration must be given to who can legally and professionally participate in providing care to the family. Nurses need to understand the professional standards and regulations which influence who can deliver care in which settings as well as associated legislation, particularly in relation to consent for treatment and guardianship, so that the options put before the family not only meet their needs but those of the legal and regulatory bodies in the country in which they reside.

Case study 5.9: Sarah

Safe care

For Frankie and his family the provision of special needs education, in and out of home care, and the maintenance of physical, cultural and psychological safe care is all influenced by the values and legal and ethical requirements of the country in which he lives. Frankie's family live in New Zealand, with cultural connections to both Maori and

(Continued)

(Continued)

Samoan cultures. Understanding and respecting the values and beliefs of the family is not only important but subject to clear codes of practice and principles within the Treaty of Waitangi in regard to protection, participation and partnership.

Frankie's family's preference for a ramp at a less visible point of access to the house was not possible because it would not meet building regulations in relation to gradients and supports, and while Frankie's parents would prefer to keep Frankie at home when he becomes unwell they recognize that, at times, safe care can only be given to him within the hospital setting.

In New Zealand it has been deemed appropriate for a non-licensed but trained carer to care for him in the home and at school when he is well. However, there are clear professional and legal boundaries in relation to what that carer can do. If Frankie requires additional treatment or care outside of the scope of this unregulated carer or his family, this may necessitate either the relocation of Frankie to a place where this care can be delivered or the introduction of additional health professionals into his home or community setting.

Although regulatory or legislative frameworks may add to the complexity of delivering care to children and families across settings, they should not be seen as a

Reflective prompts: TED 5.3

Think about whether aspects of your practice are underpinned by any beliefs, traditions or ways of working that may not be based on evidence.

- Walk around a setting where you are currently providing nursing care, e.g. hospital ward, clinic, home, community centre.
  - o Take note of the signs, labels, colours, smells, noises you encounter as you walk.
  - o Write a story, poem, reflection on what makes this environment 'home-like' or not home-like or not 'home-like'.
  - o If possible ask a child or family member to also complete the exercise.
  - o Contrast and compare those things which are 'home-like' or not 'home-like'.

Explore and evaluate the evidence, perspectives and strategies you have read in the literature and in policy and other documents.

- Consider what you have read, heard and seen and reflect on what may have influenced how the care setting has been constructed.
  - o Who is most 'at home' in this setting?
  - o Why has the environment been designed this way?

Decide, based on your reflections, how you could improve your practice. Discuss your findings with your colleagues.

- Develop a plan for how child and family spaces can be enhanced in this setting.
- What would your top three priorities be for making the environment more home-like?

barrier to child-and family-centred care. In most instances legislation and regulations exist to protect the child, family and those caring for them. Nurses can play an important role in not only the development of workable policy and legislation but also in assisting the family to understand and work within these frameworks. Nurses must be willing to advocate and negotiate on behalf of the family and to ensure legislation, policies and standards consider the needs of the families they care for.

Nurses have an important role to play in ensuring that private, shared and public spaces for children and families requiring health care are negotiated, defined and maintained, regardless of the physical location of care. Nurses caring for children and young people must recognise that the delivery of health care in whatever setting will, initially at least, be uncomfortable and impact not only on how the family functions but also on previously held understandings of privacy and home. Frequent renegotiation of private, shared and treatment spaces and how the boundaries will be traversed will need to occur as the needs of the child, family and its individual members change. Nurses have an important role to play in ensuring that health care is delivered to children and their families in safe developmentally appropriate environments which maintain all legal and regulatory standards; however, they must also recognise their advocacy role in ensuring local legislation and policy supports the needs, goals and aspirations of the families they care for.

Conclusion

This chapter has considered the increasingly diverse spaces and places in which care is delivered to children and their families and has challenged the reader to consider the impact of health care delivery on previously held understandings of family, home, private, public and communal spaces. While the increasing options available in regard to the spaces in which care is delivered can enable children's and their families' health and well-being, they can also disable, confuse and lead to tensions not only between health care provider and family but also between individual family members. This chapter has challenged the reader to think not only of the location, services and treatments to be delivered, and the physical appearance or resources required, but also the influence these may have on family functioning and the meaning the spaces and places of care may hold for children and their families.

References

Adams, A., Theodore, D., Goldenberg, E., Mclaren, C. and McKeever, P. (2010) 'Kids in the atrium: comparing architectural intentions and children's experiences in a pediatric hospital lobby', *Social Science & Medicine*, 70: 658–667.

Andrews, G.J. (2004) '(Re)thinking the dynamics between healthcare and place: therapeutic geographies in treatment and care practices', *Area*, 36: 307–318.

Andrews, G.J. and Moon, G. (2005) 'Space, place, and the evidence base: part ii – rereading nursing environment through geographical research', *Worldviews on Evidence-Based Nursing*, 2: 142–156.

Arlidge, B., Abel, S., Asiasiga, L., Milne, S.L., Crengle, S. and Ameratunga, S.N. (2009) 'Experiences of whanau/families when injured children are admitted to hospital: a multi-ethnic qualitative study from Aotearoa/New Zealand', *Ethnicity & Health*, 14: 169–183.

Avis, M. and Reardon, R. (2008) 'Understanding the views of parents of children with special needs about the nursing care their child recieves when in hospital: a qualitative study', *Journal of Child Health Care*, 12: 7–17.

Bacigalupe, G. (2011) 'Is there a role for social technologies in collaborative healthcare?', *Families, Systems & Health: The Journal of Collaborative Family Health Care*, 29: 1–14.

Bender, A., Clune, L. and Guruge, S. (2009) 'Considering place in community health nursing', *Canadian Journal of Nursing Research*, 41: 128–143.

Board, R. and Ryan-Wenger, N. (2002) 'Long-term effects of pediatric intensive care unit hospitalization on families with young children', *Heart & Lung: The Journal of Acute and Critical Care*, 31: 53–66.

Caldas, J.C.S., Pais-Ribeiro, J.L. and Carneiro, S. R. (2004) 'General anesthesia, surgery and hospitalization in children and their effects upon cognitive, academic, emotional and sociobehavioral development – a review', *Pediatric Anesthesia*, 14: 910–915.

Carnevale, F.A., Alexander, E., Davis, M., Rennick, J. and Troini, R. (2006) 'Daily living with distress and enrichment: the moral experience of families with ventilator-assisted children at home', *Pediatrics*, 117: e48–e60.

Carney, T., Murphy, S., McClure, J., Bishop, E., Kerr, C., Parker, J., Scott, F., Shields, C. and Wilson, L. (2003) 'Children's views of hospitalization: an exploratory study of data collection', *Journal of Child Health Care*, 7: 27–40.

Carter, B., Coad, J., Bray, L., Moore, A., Anderson, C., Clinchant, A., Widdas, D.Â. and Goodenough, T. (2012) 'Home-based care for special healthcare needs: community children's nursing services', *Nursing Research*, 61: 260–268.

Carter, B., Grey, J., Blake, K. and Byatt, R. (2014) '"Just kids playing sport (in a chair)": experiences of children, families and stakeholders attending a wheelchair sports club', *Disability and Sport*, doi: 10.108009687599.2014880329.

Coyne, I. (2006) 'Children's experiences of hospitalization', *Journal of Child Health Care*, 10: 326–336.

Darvill, J., Harrington, A. and Donovan, J. (2009) 'Caring for ventilated children at home: the child's perspective', *Neonatal, Paediatric and Child Health Nursing*, 12: 9–13.

Dickinson, A.R., Smythe, E. and Spence, D. (2006) 'Within the web: the family-practitioner relationship in the context of chronic childhood illness', *Journal of Child Health Care*, 10: 309–325.

Dozier, M., Zeanah, C.H., Wallin, A.R. and Shauffer, C. (2012) 'Institutional care for young children: review of literature and policy implications', *Social Issues and Policy Review*, 6: 1–25.

Earle, R.J., Rennick, J.E., Carnevale, F.A. and Davis, G.M. (2006) '"It's okay, it helps me to breathe": the experience of home ventilation from a child's perspective', *Journal of Child Health Care*, 10: 270–282.

Espezel, H.J. (2003) 'Parent-nurse interactions: care of hospitalized children', *Journal of Advanced Nursing*, 44: 34–41.

Ford, K. (2011) 'I didn't really like it, but it sounded exciting', *Journal of Child Health Care*, 15: 250–260.

Gilmour, J.A. (2006) 'Hybrid space: constituting the hospital as a home space for patients', *Nursing Inquiry*, 13: 16–22.

Gray, J.E., Safran, C., Davis, R.B., Pompilio-Weitzner, G., Stewart, J.E., Zaccagnini, L. and Pursley, D. (2000) 'Baby CareLink: using the internet and telemedicine to improve care for high-risk infants', *Pediatrics*, 106: 1318–1324.

Hall, W. and Irvine, V. (2009) 'E-communication among mothers of infants and toddlers in a community-based cohort: a content analysis', *Journal of Advanced Nursing*, 65: 175–183.

Health and Disability Commissioner (2009) *The Act and Code*. New Zealand: Health and Disabiity Commissioner. Available at: www.hdc.org.nz/the-act--code (accessed 19 May 2013).

Heaton, J., Noyes, J., Sloper, P. and Shah, R. (2005) 'Families' experiences of caring for technology-dependent children: a temporal perspective', *Health & Social Care in the Community*, 13: 441–450.

Hinckson, E.A., Dickinson, A., Water, T., Sands, M. and Penman, L. (2013) 'Physical activity, dietary habits and overall health in overweight and obese children and youth with intellectual disability or autism', *Research in Developmental Disabilities*, 34: 1170–1178.

Hopia, H., Tomlinson, P.S., Paavilainen, E. and Åstedt-Kurki, P. (2005) 'Child in hospital: family experiences and expectations of how nurses can promote family health', *Journal of Clinical Nursing*, 14: 212–222.

Huang, I.C., Sugden, D. and Beveridge, S. (2009) 'Children's perceptions of their use of assistive devices in home and school settings', *Disability and Rehabilitation: Assistive Technology*, 4: 95–105.

Hutton, A. (2005) 'Consumer perspectives in adolescent ward design', *Journal of Clinical Nursing*, 14: 537–545.

Imms, C., Reilly, S., Carlin, J. and Dodd, K.J. (2009) 'Characteristics influencing participation of Australian children with cerebral palsy', *Disability & Rehabilitation*, 31: 2204–2215.

Johnson, R., Browne, K. and Hamilton-Giachritsis, C. (2006) 'Young children in institutional care at risk of harm', *Trauma, Violence, & Abuse*, 7: 34–60.

Kearns, R.A. and Barnett, J.R. (2000) '"Happy Meals" in the Starship Enterprise: interpreting a moral geography of health care consumption', *Health & Place*, 6: 81–93.

Kearns, R.A. and Collins, D.C.A. (2000) 'New Zealand children's health camps: therapeutic landscapes meet the contract state', *Social Science & Medicine*, 51: 1047–1059.

Kholen, C., Beier, J. and Danzer, G. (2000) '"They don't leave you on your own": a qualitative study of the home care of chronically ill children', *Pediatric Nursing*, 26: 364–371.

Kirk, S. (2010) 'How children and young people construct and negotiate living with medical technology', *Social Science & Medicine*, 71: 1796–1803.

Malone, R.E. (2003) 'Distal nursing', *Social Science & Medicine*, 56: 2317–2326.

McConkey, R., Nixon, T., Donaghy, E. and Mulhern, D. (2004) 'The characteristics of children with a disability looked after away from home and their future service needs', *British Journal of Social Work*, 34: 561–576.

McKeever, P., O'Neill, S. and Miller, K.-L. (2002) 'Managing space and marking time: mothering severely ill infants in hospital isolation', *Qualitative Health Research*, 12: 1020–1032.

Milligan, C. (2003) 'Location or dis-location? Towards a conceptualization of people and place in the care-giving experience', *Social & Cultural Geography*, 4: 455–470.

Mirfin-Veitch, B., Bray, A. and Ross, N. (2003) '"It was the hardest and most painful decision of my life!": seeking permanent out-of-home placement for sons and daughters with intellectual disabilities', *Journal of Intellectual & Developmental Disability*, 28: 99–111.

Moore, A.J., Anderson, C., Carter, B. and Coad, J. (2010) 'Appropriated landscapes: the intrusion of technology and equipment into the homes and lives of families with a child with complex needs', *Journal of Child Health Care*, 14: 3–5.

Moore, A.J. and Carter, B. (2012) 'The place of assistive technologies in the homes and lives of families with a child with complex healthcare needs', *Environmental and Architectural Phenomenology*, 23 (2): 11–14

Peter, E. and Liaschenko, J. (2004) 'Perils of proximity: a spatiotemporal analysis of moral distress and moral ambiguity', *Nursing Inquiry*, 11: 218–225.

Poland, B., Lehoux, P., Holmes, D. and Andrews, G. (2005) 'How place matters: unpacking technology and power in health and social care', *Health & Social Care in the Community*, 13: 170–180.

Sellick, C. (1998) 'The use of institutional care for children across Europe', *European Journal of Social Work*, 1: 301–310.

Smith, A. (2007) 'Telemedicine: challenges and opportunities', *Expert Rev. Med. Devices*, 4: 5–7.

Smith-Stoner, M. (2011) 'Webcasting in home and hospice care services', *Home Healthcare Nurse*, 29: 337–341.

Vickers, J., Thompson, A., Collins, G.S., Childs, M. and Hain, R. (2007) 'Place and provision of palliative care for children with progressive cancer: a study by the Paediatric Oncology Nurses' Forum/United Kingdom Children's Cancer Study Group Palliative Care Working Group', *Journal of Clinical Oncology*, 25: 4472–4476.

Vickers, J.L. and Carlisle, C. (2000) 'Choices and control: parental experiences in pediatric terminal home care', *Journal of Pediatric Oncology Nursing*, 17: 12–21.

Wilson, H.V. (2001) 'Power and partnership: a crtical analysis of the surveillance discourses of child health nurses', *Journal of Advanced Nursing*, 36: 294–301.

Yantzi, N.M., Rosenberg, M.W. and McKeever, P. (2007) 'Getting out of the house: the challenges mothers face when their children have long-term care needs', *Health & Social Care in the Community*, 15: 45–55.

Young, N.L., Barden, W., McKeever, P., Dick, P.T. and Tele-Homecare Team (2006) 'Taking the call-bell home: a qualitative evaluation of Tele-Home Care for children', *Health & Social Care in the Community*, 14: 231–241.

Chapter 6

Understanding Children's and Young People's Experiences of Illness

Key points

- Children and young people experience a range of illnesses and symptoms.
- Children's and young people's understanding of illness is dependent upon many factors including age, experience, personality and cognitive ability.
- Children's and young people's concerns about being ill are different to those of adults.
- Both being ill and being in hospital can make children and young people feel vulnerable and provoke fear.
- Illness and treatment impacts upon children's and young peoples' lives and can feel all encompassing.

Key theories and concepts explored in this chapter are illness, symptoms and treatment.

Case study 6.1: Harry

Setting the scene

Harry is 5 years old and lives at home with his parents and brother, aged six months. Over the past three years he has been suffering from recurrent throat infections necessitating frequent courses of oral antibiotics. After being seen by his GP he is referred to the ENT surgeon at the local hospital and put on the waiting list to undergo a tonsillectomy. Harry's mother is anxious about him having to go into hospital as he has been increasingly dependent on her since the birth of his brother. Her partner works long hours away from home resulting in her being the main carer and she is worried about providing care for both children while Harry is in hospital.

Introduction

Children experience being ill as part of growing up and learning about themselves and the world they live in. For many children the common diseases of childhood, such as coughs and colds, are relatively minor and recovered from quickly without long-term effects. However, this is largely dependent on their health and robustness beforehand and whether there are underlying factors such as poverty, malnutrition or other morbidities. Globally, many differences exist in terms of the under-5 mortality rate and burden of disease; 14 African countries have noted deteriorating child mortality rates in the last 10 years (United Nations 2007). Infants and children in India, for example, are more likely to die of a preventable or treatable childhood illness than their counterparts in developed countries. Meanwhile, specific diseases are more prevalent in certain countries, for example Human Immunodeficiency Virus (HIV) in Africa and rheumatic fever in New Zealand. Depending on the definitions and measures used, variability exists within the prevalence figures for children living with disability (Carter 2014); within the United Kingdom this is estimated as 800,000 children (The Children's Society 2011) and globally approximately 200 million children (Lansdown 2009).

As was noted in Chapter 1, children and young people experience illness and disability differently to adults. The range of illnesses they experience is vast and symptoms can arise from all systems, such as seizures from epilepsy and respiratory symptoms from asthma or bronchiolitis. Children have to face illness and symptoms often with less capacity, understanding and control than adults, although the symptoms are just as overwhelming and difficult to deal with. Coupled with a developing cognitive understanding, children's imagination can result in them experiencing things very differently to the way in which adults may appreciate. Being admitted to hospital or visiting the doctor often incurs fears and concerns about being in unknown and unfamiliar settings and situations. However, as children experience illness and its associated symptoms they start to understand more about their bodies, health and being ill. The way that they are cared for and responded to is vital in promoting a positive experience. This chapter considers children's and young people's experiences of illness and symptoms and the ways in which these impact upon children and young people themselves and their families.

Children's and young people's understanding of illness

As children grow they learn about illness, both as part of the maturation process and as they, and others they know, experience ill health. Children's and young people's understanding of illness is affected by factors such as age (Forsner et al. 2005a), the influences of family, culture, cognitive and linguistic ability, experience and personality (Moules and Ramsay 2008). For example, pre-school children often accept what they are told about illness and may interpret literally what is said (Moules and Ramsay 2008), while some children under the age of 7 years may associate illness with misbehaviour. School-age children may develop an understanding of the consequences of illness which can lead to frustration when it limits their abilities (Moules and Ramsay 2008). At this stage, information sharing enables children to cope better with illness and hospitalisation and many children with long-term illness have been shown to be able to share their important perspectives (Edwards 2009). For adolescents, being ill and/or in hospital increases their dependence on others and results in them experiencing a loss of control (Edwards 2009). This may impact greatly upon them at a time when they are beginning to develop independence. At this age adolescents are aware of potential issues around illness and treatment and wish to be fully informed (Edwards, 2009).

The ways in which children view health can affect how information about illness is interpreted. For example, children may be reluctant to take medicine for pain if they do not understand how this will relieve their headache. Similarly, children may have vivid images about undergoing surgery or specific procedures. Research has shown that for many children and young people having injections or needles is one of their greatest fears when in hospital (Coyne 2006).

Case study 6.2: Harry

Having an operation

Harry is worried about going into hospital. He wonders if it is because he has been naughty. He has been having nightmares about his forthcoming operation, dreaming that the nurses will give him injections that will hurt. His friend at school has told him that the doctor will have to cut his throat wide open to take his tonsils out. Harry wishes that he did not have to have the operation and that he could make Mum change her mind about it.

Historically, academic consideration of children's understanding of illness has relied heavily upon Piaget's theory of cognitive development, arguably the most accepted and absolute image of childhood to be encountered in the Western world (James et al. 2001). This perspective, based on natural growth and viewing development in terms of a progression, perceives age and competence as intertwined with, and determined by, the development of the child's body. However, this theory has been increasingly challenged, with writers suggesting that young children have more understanding than implied by Piaget's theory (Meadows 1993) and that Piaget's ideal of adult cognitive competence is peculiarly Western and culture bound (Archard 1993). While the field of developmental psychology itself acknowledges the failure of the theory to take account of the impact of social and cultural contexts on the development of children (Woodhead 1997), sociologists of childhood have criticised its focus on age-related competencies, resulting in an impoverished understanding of what it means to be a child (Hogan 2006). The application of Piaget's approach to children's understanding of illness has been questioned (Sigelman et al. 1993), with studies revealing that children with a chronic illness have a greater and different understanding of illness than those without (Crisp et al. 1996). For example, children with asthma acknowledge their illness as potentially fatal with a risk of dying from a lack of air (Yoos and McMullen 1996). While for many children and young people increasing age is commensurate with cognitive and physical development and growing independence, this may not be the case for those with cognitive impairment or long-term complex needs where dependence upon others may continue or even increase as their condition progresses. As a result, Piaget's theory precludes these important groups. Thus, an approach which considers the interplay of culture and past experiences of hospital and illness may better represent children's and young people's understanding of being ill.

While it has been acknowledged that health service professionals may limit children's participation in discussing important or potentially upsetting issues under the guise of protecting them (Berman 2003), studies have shown that children and young people across cultures prefer to be told about their illness rather than fear the unknown (Bunn 2010; CLIC Sargent 2010). The distress caused by illness requires a highly skilled response from professionals who understand and are trained in the unique needs of children and adolescents (The Paediatric Society of New Zealand 2002). It is important that nurses are able to communicate effectively with children and young people, providing information about their illness and treatment in ways they can understand, whilst ascertaining and addressing their particular fears. For children and young people with limited verbal or cognitive ability, liaising with parents who are the experts on their child's understanding and communication methods may reveal the best way to share information regarding their illness and treatment with them in order to ensure they do not feel isolated and afraid.

In summary, children's and young people's understanding of illness develops with both age and exposure to illness and is affected by many influences, including family and personality. The ways in which children and young people view health can impact upon how illness and its treatment are interpreted. Children may have vivid images about surgery and undergoing treatment, particularly having needles or injections. Consequently, nurses have an important role in understanding the ways in which children and young people of different ages view and interpret illness in order to effectively address their fears.

Experiences of being ill

When considering experiences of illness it is important to consider the impact of these experiences on children, young people and families. Traditionally, children's and young people's experiences of illness have been investigated through the eyes of parents and professionals, reflecting the assumption that the perspectives of children and young people can best be elicited from adults (Docherty and Sandelowski 1999). However, it has been argued that illness can have different meanings for different people, with patients often holding a subjective, emotional view and professionals basing their understanding around objective symptoms (Forsner et al. 2005a). Children and young people are concerned about different aspects of being ill to adults and past studies suggest that the accounts of adults, extensively used as proxies for children and young people, may not accurately reflect the perceptions of children and young people themselves (Battrick and Glasper 2004; Chesney et al. 2005; Lumeng et al. 2001). Illness can cause disruption to children's and young people's normal lives (Forsner et al. 2005b) and to their sense of well-being (Coyne 2006), while treatments in hospital may render them powerless and further dependent upon their parents or nurses (Edwards 2009). However, this is not to say that this reflects upon children's and young people's everyday normal capacities and capabilities and that they are passive within their illness experience.

As previously mentioned, children and young people experience a vast range of illnesses, some are acute and short term while others are chronic and life-long. Some diseases necessitate medical treatment and even technological intervention for many years or over the course of a lifetime (Hewitt-Taylor 2008), while others may be life threatening and result in a need for critical intervention and therapy. Throughout the illness experience, children and young people may be fragile and vulnerable both physiologically and psychologically, with their responses to illness differing from those of adults (The Paediatric Society of New Zealand 2002).

While perceptions of living with a chronic long-term illness and having a child with complex and/or continuing care needs have been widely researched, children's and young people's perspectives of acute short-term illness have received much less attention. However, the experiences of children and young people with cancer and those of their parents have been extensively explored, and the nature of this range of diseases as acute initially, yet potentially chronic and life threatening, make their perceptions and experiences transferrable to a range of other illnesses and situations. This chapter will consider children's and young people's experiences from these differing perspectives.

Case study 6.3: Harry

Being ill

Harry hated having sore throats all the time. Even though his teacher at school said 'it was only a sore throat', sometimes he felt so poorly that he couldn't sleep, or play with his friends or even eat his favourite tea. It made him feel sad to be poorly so much.

Being ill: acute illness

For most children and young people, admission to hospital is as a result of a short-term, acute illness. For children with an acute illness, falling ill can come as 'a bolt from the blue' (Forsner et al. 2005a: 161) with children describing feeling trapped and talking of pain, frightening experiences and thoughts (Forsner et al. 2005a). Similarly, young people may see the disruption of short-term illness as a surprise, with little time to adjust (Forsner et al. 2005b); their lack of experience of illness may influence their perspectives, resulting in them feeling lost and uncertain of what to expect. Some illnesses, such as asthma and diabetes mellitus, can be chronic and yet have exacerbations that are acute and can be life threatening. Figure 6.1 illustrates the limitations and restrictions of having asthma from the perspective of a 7-year-old when invited to draw a picture to depict her feelings about being ill (Edwards 2009).

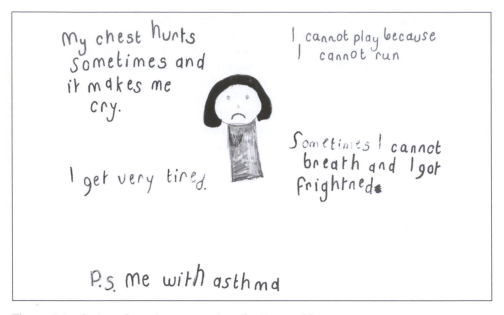

Figure 6.1   Asthma from the perspective of a 7-year-old

Her drawing, portraying her as looking sad, incorporated her feelings about the restrictions having asthma imposed upon her. On talking about her picture, she described not being able to play with her friends due to feeling very tired and becoming breathless and the way in which this led her to feel frightened when she felt she was struggling to breathe.

Being ill: having cancer

After accidents, cancer is the leading cause of death in children, with more than 160,000 children diagnosed worldwide each year (International Children's Palliative Care Network (ICPCN) 2012). Every day 10 families in the UK are told their child has cancer (CLIC Sargent 2011) with more than 10,000 children and young people receiving treatment at any time (CLIC Sargent 2011). With significant advances in treatment methods, childhood cancer in developed countries can now be viewed as a chronic and, life threatening illness rather than a disease that is incurable (Stewart 2003; Wong and Chan 2006). However, with 80% of the children diagnosed living in developing countries, it is anticipated that more than half will die through a lack of access to early detection, treatment and care (International Children's Palliative Care Network (ICPCN) 2012).

Childhood cancer therapy is characterised by repetitive episodes of intensive treatment and while this offers legitimate hope for a cure, therapy is unpredictable. Relapse, long-term toxicity and even death from illness or treatment adds to the unpredictability of the disease, thus creating a 'paradox of increased optimism accompanied by enduring uncertainty' (Stewart 2003: 394). Consequently, it has been argued that the ambiguity of outcome in severe childhood illnesses is best understood within the framework of uncertainty (Jessop and Stein 1985), with the Sword of Damocles being used to depict the pervasive threat of relapse, death and long-term effects.

Children's and young people's experiences of cancer are described within three categories; physical, emotional and social (CLIC Sargent 2010). The emotional impact of being diagnosed with cancer and undergoing treatment greatly impacts upon children's social worlds, resulting in them being different both in physical appearance and in the ways in which others treat them (CLIC Sargent 2010). Children report concern that being ill often results in symptoms leading to a loss of ability to function as normal and this impacts upon all parts of daily living. However, despite the enormity of childhood cancer and its life changing impact, children place emphasis on viewing their lives as ordinary and routine despite undergoing extensive treatment (Stewart 2003). This view concurs with studies of children with chronic illness which note the importance of striving for normalcy (Admi 1996; Atkin and Ahmad 2001; Christian and D'Auria 1997; Horner 1999; Wise 2002). At the time of diagnosis, young people have reported fearing alienation, altered appearance, medical treatments and dying (Hedstrom et al. 2004). However, they also identified that knowledge is preferable to uncertainty, expressing both hope to recover and the relief of having a diagnosis (Hedstrom et al. 2004). Socially, young people with cancer have reported feeling isolated, with education priorities often changing due to the effects of treatment and limited future work prospects (CLIC Sargent 2011).

Whilst the diagnosis of a malignant disease can be overwhelming for an adult, societal norms about childhood make it a particularly harrowing diagnosis for families. The death of a child defies the expected natural order of life events (Sourkes et al. 2005), making potentially fatal illnesses in children difficult for families to come to terms with. The diagnosis of childhood cancer has been identified as a 'pivotal turning point' (Woodgate 2006: 6), fracturing the reality of children's and families' lives (Clarke-Steffen 1993) and changing the course of their lives forever (Woodgate 2006). Cancer, as a phenomenon, requires families to not only embark on an uncertain and exhausting journey but also to confront the possible death of their child (Comaroff and Maguire 1981; Sterken 1996). In the midst of the emotional turbulence of diagnosis; denial, normalisation and participation have been identified as the main strategies used by parents to deal with their child's illness (Forinder 2004). Shock and denial, establishing the meaning of the situation, confronting the reality and establishing a new perspective have been reported by Chinese parents (Wong and Chan 2006).

Being ill: chronic illness and complex and/or continuing care needs

Chronic illnesses have been defined as those that affect children for extended periods of time, often for life, and which can be managed in terms of symptom control but not cured (Eiser 1990). Children and young people with chronic illnesses may experience uncertainty regarding their illness (Atkin and Ahmad 2001) and concerns around the perceptions and attitudes of others (Rhee et al. 2007). The limitations imposed by illness and treatment and feelings of being different (Eklund and Sivberg 2003) resonate across experiences. For instance, children and young people with type 1 diabetes mellitus have identified difference through living with diabetes and the visibility of their pursuit of 'normal' (Marshall 2010; Marshall et al. 2009), while children with asthma strive to live normal lives (Rydstrom et al. 1999). The dominance of, and restrictions incurred by, chronic illness are also widely acknowledged. Work exploring the experiences of children and young people with long-term renal illness has vividly described the ways in which illness dominates their lives, describing children living and growing up in a 'renal space' (the haemodialysis unit) and living in a renal body (Lindsay Waters 2008). Children and young people themselves have also identified the restrictions imposed by chronic illness and the domination of daily routines necessary to manage illness (Edwards 2009).

The diagnosis of chronic illness in children has been described as a cataclysmic event, shattering parents' worlds (Cohen 1993; Massie and Massie 1975) and launching them into unchartered territory (Steele 2005). While the ways in which caring for children and young people with acute, chronic and complex illnesses impacts upon parents and families will be elaborated upon later in this chapter, it is important to note here the demands made upon parents, with mothers in particular experiencing stress related to the consequences and demands of caring for a child with chronic illness (Young et al. 2002).

Continuing improvements in medical care has led to a growing number of children with complex and/or continuing care needs (Department of Health 2004). While there is no absolute definition of a complex health need (Stalker et al. 2003), increasing numbers of children and young people may remain dependent on technology for sustained periods of time (Kirk 1999). Technology dependent children have been defined as those who 'have dependence on a technological device to sustain life or optimise health and have the need for substantial and complex nursing care for substantial parts of the day or night' (Glendinning et al. 1999: 35), including dependence on gastrostomy or naso-gastric feeding equipment, oxygen, suction, tracheostomy and ventilator support (Beale 2002).

While some similarities exist, the unique issues families with a technologically dependent child face, over and above those of a chronically ill child, include a lengthy initial hospital stay, greater parental stress, financial burden, the need to share homes with equipment and health professionals, delays in discharge, inadequate service provision, cost shifting (Darvill et al. 2009) and disparity to services (Noyes 2000).

Despite children and young people with complex and/or continuing care needs often requiring frequent and prolonged hospital stays, emphasis is now placed on care that is home based (Department of Health 2011; Milligan and Whiles 2010). Where children and young people are dependent upon medical equipment and complicated therapies and routines, parents have to manage sophisticated technology and interventions in order to meet their needs (Carter 2005; Carter et al. 2011), leading to family life revolving around technology and care routines. As a result, homes become medicalised with necessary equipment, supplies and the presence of carers or professionals (Kirk et al. 2005; Moore et al. 2010). Caring for a child with complex and/or continuing care needs has been identified as impacting physically, psychologically, emotionally, spiritually and environmentally upon children and their families (Moore et al. 2010), with fatigue, depression and isolation being identified (MacDonald and Callery 2007; McCallin et al. 2007). Parents have reported an overwhelming responsibility towards their ventilator-dependent child and significant emotional, physical and psychological strain (Carnevale et al. 2006). Their role in caring for a child with complex and/or continuing care needs has been depicted as one that begins from birth and continues indefinitely, revealing the overwhelming situation parents find themselves in (MacDonald and Callery 2007); while families of children with disabilities can feel marginalised (Lyons et al. 2009).

In summary, children and young people experience a vast range of illnesses, some acute and short term, others chronic and lasting for long periods of time and some life limiting or threatening. Children and young people with acute illness may have pain and frightening thoughts and experiences alongside feeling trapped, while those with chronic illnesses have described the restrictions imposed by their illness and the ways in which being ill dominates their lives. For parents of children with complex and/or continuing care needs, the incessant demands and onerous responsibility placed upon them in providing care to their child pervade their accounts. It is essential for nurses to acknowledge these varied experiences of illness and to ensure that children's and young people's differing needs are met.

Being in hospital

As reported in Chapter 1, historically hospitals were miserable places for children and young people, where they were not allowed to play but expected to lie quietly, with family only permitted to visit infrequently (The Paediatric Society of New Zealand, 2002). In a paper entitled *Hospital: A Deprived Environment for Children?* (Save the Children 1989: 31) it was recommended that 'the emotional and psychological needs of children must be afforded a priority equal to that of their physical needs in order that immediate distress and/or long term behavioural or psychiatric disturbance may be avoided'. It has been argued that little progress has been made in addressing the emotional and psychological needs of children in hospital, with Southall et al. (2000) noting that while modern medical technology and treatment regimens have improved the survival rates of sick children, commensurate attention has not always been paid to the fear, distress and suffering they experience while undergoing treatment or care in a health care facility. Still more recently, children's stories about being in hospital describe feelings of being alone, 'scared, mad and sad' (Wilson et al. 2010).

While admission to hospital and undergoing surgery or medical procedures can be unpleasant for adults, it is recognised that unique factors exist for children. Being in hospital can disrupt the lives of children and young people in terms of their everyday routines (Wise 2002). Taking children and young people out of their familiar everyday environments and putting them into the unfamiliar hospital setting erodes any power bases they may have and increases their dependence on others. Many children may feel scared and fearful of the unknown (Fletcher et al. 2011), while distress at being separated from parents, siblings and friends within the unfamiliar hospital setting may further increase anxiety (Coyne 2006). Children in hospital are often vulnerable due to their illness and have little control over events happening to them (Bricher 2000), resulting in a loss of control and increasing their dependence (Coyne 2003, 2006). It is important to acknowledge that some children may associate admission to hospital as a means of chastisement. Children with pervasive developmental disorder have described punishment and persecution as the main constructs to explain hospitalisation (Stefanatou 2008).

As discussed in Chapter 1, it is now widely acknowledged that the presence of parents and family during children's and young people's admission to hospital ameliorates the adverse effects experienced, while minimising distress and accelerating recovery (Kennedy 2001). This is corroborated by studies highlighting that both parental presence and support from nursing staff help children cope with anxiety around separation (LeRoy et al. 2003; Rennick et al. 2004), with the presence of and support from parents and family being particularly important (Ford 2011). Crucially, research with children themselves has also demonstrated the importance of parental presence during hospitalisation (Carney et al. 2003; Salmela et al. 2010). Parental presence is now widely stipulated in a number of guidelines (Department of Health 2004; The Paediatric Society of New Zealand 2002), and it is acknowledged that a child should only be admitted to hospital if the care they require cannot be provided at home (Royal College of Nursing (RCN) 2011; The Paediatric Society of New Zealand 2002).

Case study 6.4: Harry

Going into hospital

Harry remains worried about having to go into hospital. He knows that Mum is worried about him – she cried when the doctor said he needed an operation – and he is frightened that there is something she is not telling him. He is scared that no one will be able to visit or stay with him while he is in hospital, especially now he has his little brother. Before it was just him, Mum and Dad but now the baby always seems to come before him. He wishes things were as they used to be.

For some children and young people, their illness or the effects of treatment may necessitate the need for critical intervention and therapy resulting in admission to a Paediatric Intensive Care Unit (PICU) or High Dependency Unit (HDU). Intensive care units carry a multitude of equipment, amidst a cacophony of noise. For recovering children and young people, the PICU can evoke anxiety both for themselves and for others. One young person in a study exploring children's and young people's perspectives of being in hospital (Edwards 2009: 157) vividly described her experiences of being in this setting:

One lad was brought in on an ambulance stretcher. You know the ambulance crew actually brought him up. He looked in a right bad way. I think he'd been in a car accident or something. He was strapped on to the stretcher and you could see tubes everywhere. His mum and dad came in and they were crying when they saw him. His mum ran off when she saw him. ... It's scary you know on intensive care. I think it's all the equipment everywhere and the nurses rushing about. ... It really scared me when the lad was brought in. It was the middle of the night and I was lying in the next bed while everyone was rushing about and I was thinking how sick he looked. It really scared me. I thought he's only a lad. He's even younger than me. What if he dies or something? I could tell that all the nurses were worried about him. I could tell by the looks on their faces and the way that they were rushing around. You know, two doctors were by him all night and that doesn't happen unless something is really wrong. I just laid there and felt really worried for him. And for his mum and dad too. ... And I thought please don't let him die. Not here in the bed next to me.

Parents meanwhile have recounted catastrophic feelings of confusion, helplessness, shock, guilt and crisis when their child is admitted to a PICU, describing this setting as strange and daunting (Noyes 1999). When considering how families

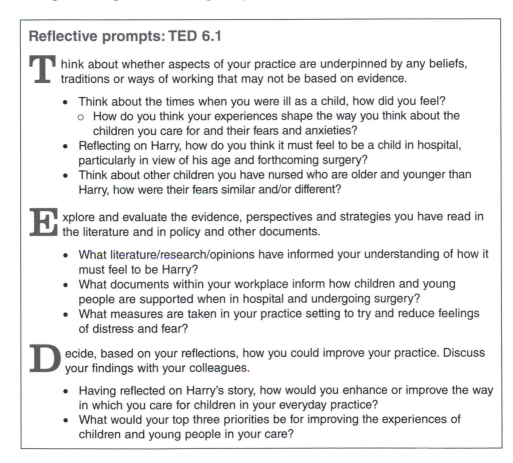

Reflective prompts: TED 6.1

Think about whether aspects of your practice are underpinned by any beliefs, traditions or ways of working that may not be based on evidence.

- Think about the times when you were ill as a child, how did you feel?
  - How do you think your experiences shape the way you think about the children you care for and their fears and anxieties?
- Reflecting on Harry, how do you think it must feel to be a child in hospital, particularly in view of his age and forthcoming surgery?
- Think about other children you have nursed who are older and younger than Harry, how were their fears similar and/or different?

Explore and evaluate the evidence, perspectives and strategies you have read in the literature and in policy and other documents.

- What literature/research/opinions have informed your understanding of how it must feel to be Harry?
- What documents within your workplace inform how children and young people are supported when in hospital and undergoing surgery?
- What measures are taken in your practice setting to try and reduce feelings of distress and fear?

Decide, based on your reflections, how you could improve your practice. Discuss your findings with your colleagues.

- Having reflected on Harry's story, how would you enhance or improve the way in which you care for children in your everyday practice?
- What would your top three priorities be for improving the experiences of children and young people in your care?

may experience their child being admitted to PICU the following description is vivid: 'culturally recognisable ideas of children as being "full of life" are dramatically transformed. In the PICU (Paediatric Intensive Care Unit) they lie immobilised, at the boundary of life and death' (Place 2000: 172).

Perhaps unsurprisingly, it is acknowledged that admission to intensive care carries a higher risk of psychological and behavioural problems for children than those cared for within the general ward setting (Jones et al. 1992). Anxiety, helplessness and depression have also been identified in parents of children and young people who have been cared for in the intensive care unit setting (Board 2005), with stress-related symptoms persisting in mothers as long as six months after their child's illness, indicating the trauma of a child's illness and admission to intensive care (Board and Ryan-Wenger 2002).

In summary, the detrimental effects incurred by hospitalisation have been widely reported, with children and young people experiencing powerlessness and disruption in the hospital setting and anxiety around being separated from those important to them. The importance of parental and family presence is widely acknowledged and it is recognised that this both reduces the adverse effects experienced and increases recovery time. It is essential for nurses to have an awareness of the fears experienced by children and young people while in hospital and to attempt to address these.

Perceptions of treatment and symptoms

Children and young people experience a wide variety of illnesses and symptoms necessitating many different types of treatment and procedures. It is now widely acknowledged that children experience heightened anxiety around undergoing surgery (Ford 2011), including fear around the surgical journey itself, investigations (Coyne 2006), taking medications and receiving injections (Edwards 2009), with symptoms of illness and undergoing procedures and treatment cited as amongst the worst aspects of being in hospital (Pelander and Leino-Kilpi 2010). This chapter will consider children's and young people's perceptions of treatment and symptoms.

Undergoing treatment

It has been demonstrated that children in hospital experience procedure-related pain (Drendel et al. 2006; Nilsson et al. 2009) during nursing, medical and diagnostic procedures. This may relate to examinations, investigations and/or the administration of medications and treatments (Kortesluoma and Nikkonen 2004), including needles and intravenous lines (Franck et al. 2008). Venepuncture has been described as one of the 'worst kinds of pain' (Kortesluoma and Nikkonen 2004: 219), with pain during and following infusions of medications or blood products the most intense (Kortesluoma and Nikkonen 2004). Seeing the instruments to be used in a procedure increased the intensity of the pain experienced by children (Kortesluoma and Nikkonen 2004).

Not surprisingly, the pain related to the therapeutic and diagnostic procedures experienced by children can be associated with substantial anxiety and stress (Ortiz et al. 2012) while those procedures that health care professionals deem to be routine or minor can be momentous for children and their families (Ford et al. 2012). It has been reported that children in hospital find ordinary nursing interventions frightening and even traumatic (Salmela et al. 2010), describing fear and anxiety from diagnostics procedures such as radiography, sonography and blood sampling (Bjorkman et al. 2012; Bsiri-Moghaddam et al. 2011). Indeed, children have described fears related to nursing procedures and pain as amongst the worst aspects of being in hospital (Carney et al. 2003).

For those children undergoing surgery, pre-operative preparation programmes are recognised as one way of reducing anxiety in children (Buckley and Savage, 2010), with those receiving preparation demonstrating less fear and expressing more understanding and acknowledgement of their surgical procedure than those who received none (Teixeira and de Figueiredo 2009). On questioning, children between 7 and 17 years undergoing surgery indicated a desire for information about pain and anaesthesia, procedures and potential complications (Fortier et al. 2009; Smith and Callery 2005), while children aged between 6 and 9 years undergoing tonsillectomy described a need for pre-operative information around the operative procedure, soreness and discomfort post-operatively and parental presence (Buckley and Savage 2010).

Case study 6.5: Harry

Having an operation

Harry is very worried about having an operation. He is scared that when the doctor makes him go to sleep he might not wake up afterwards. Someone at school told him that he will have to have a big needle that will hurt a lot and he once saw a hospital programme on television where a man was really poorly and he had to have lots of needles. He hopes that won't happen to him.

Children and young people have described treatment in hospital as being relentless and permeating their hospital stay (Edwards 2009) and this is graphically revealed in the activity report of one young person of a typical day in hospital, demonstrating the incessant nature of treatment regimens and the way in which the daily management of her illness virtually dominates her whole day (see Figure 6.2).

For children and young people with cancer, treatment can be lengthy, with potential side effects, complications, painful procedures and treatments (Hedstrom et al. 2004). The 'daunting nature of therapy' in terms of sleeping, nausea, vomiting, mood swings and the ways in which 'the practicalities of life became almost insurmountable' have

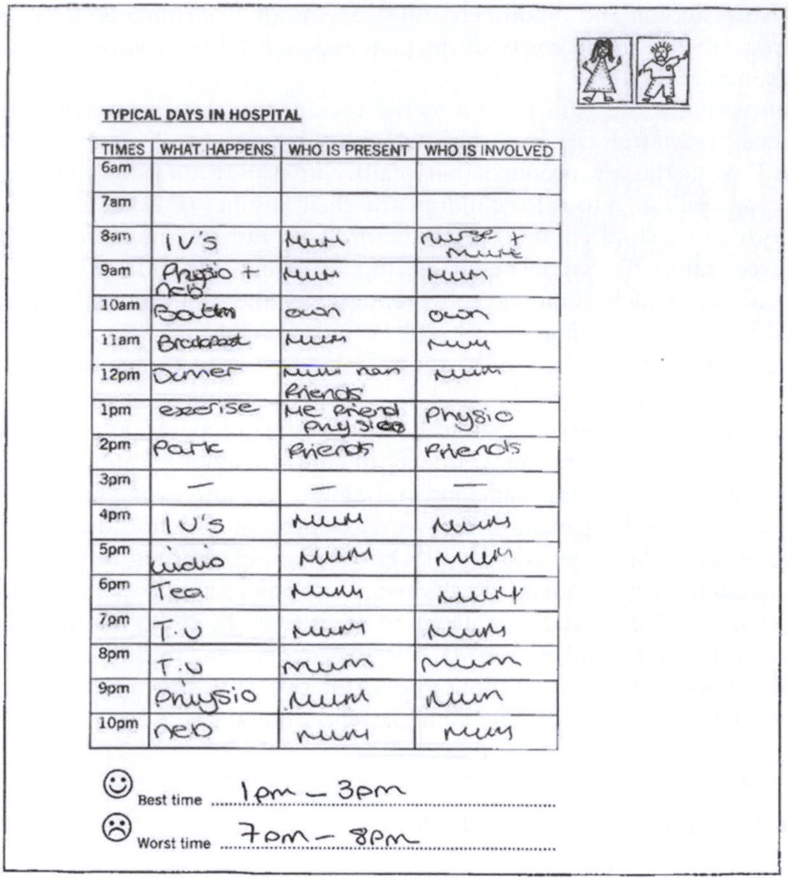

TYPICAL DAYS IN HOSPITAL

TIMES	WHAT HAPPENS	WHO IS PRESENT	WHO IS INVOLVED
6am			
7am			
8am	IV's	Mum	nurse + mum
9am	Physio + neb	Mum	Mum
10am	Bath	own	own
11am	Breakfast	Mum	Mum
12pm	Dinner	Mum nan friends	Mum
1pm	exercise	Me friend physio	Physio
2pm	Park	friends	friends
3pm	—	—	—
4pm	IV's	Mum	Mum
5pm	Video	Mum	Mum
6pm	Tea	Mum	Mum
7pm	T.V	Mum	Mum
8pm	T.V	mum	mum
9pm	Physio	Mum	Mum
10pm	neb	Mum	Mum

Best time 1pm – 3pm

Worst time 7pm – 8pm

Figure 6.2 A chart of a typical day in hospital for one young person

been vividly described, alongside the effect on psychological well-being in terms of nightmares, stress and 'scary' illness and treatment (Gibson et al. 2005: 656). Children have described how illness and treatment places limitations on their lives when feeling tired and sick, with older children reporting feeling worried about the present and future, particularly in relation to whether they would get better. From children's and young people's perspective, the effects of taking medications routinely, daily injections and the application of creams are all encompassing, leaving little time for having fun (CLIC Sargent 2010). Children highlight the visible side effects of treatment, including hair loss associated with chemotherapy and the facial bloating and puffiness associated with steroid therapy, as singling them out as different to others (Bluebond-Langner 1978; CLIC Sargent 2010). This may be of particular significance to older children and adolescents where physical appearance and peer pressure is particularly important. The most distressing aspects of receiving chemotherapy for adolescents are altered self-image, including hair loss, fatigue, loss of appetite and weight; feeling confined by being attached to intravenous lines and naso-gastric tubes and physical concerns around nausea, vomiting, mouth ulcers and pain (Hedstrom et al. 2003, 2004). Understandably, children with cancer revealed a dislike of undergoing treatment, preferring it to be kept as short as possible and with few side effects (CLIC Sargent 2010). Children also report concerns about mortality, particularly in children who had experienced the death of a friend.

Being at a more susceptible stage of cognitive, biological and psychological development means that young people are likely to be hit harder by the side effects caused by therapy; problems secondary to treatment are well documented (Forinder and Posse 2008). Indeed, the physical and mental effects of treatment may impact upon children, young people and parents for many years following its end. On-going mental distress has been identified in young people years after stem cell transplantation, with the physical effects of treatment being cited as a significant contributing factor (Forinder and Posse 2008). From the perspective of parents of children undergoing stem cell transplantation, the heavy demands that the treatment had on both themselves and their child and the dilemmas faced in terms of the potential side effects of the treatment were significant (Forinder 2004). While the stem cell procedure posed a threat involving potentially dangerous consequences, several parents saw it as a 'straw to grasp' (Forinder 2004: 139). Fears around losing their child were heightened during the transplant, and anxiety in regard to the long-term effects on their child persisted for up to four to eight years following treatment.

Experiencing symptoms

The distress of symptoms and an inability to manage these can cause suffering for children and families (Kim and Morrow 2003; McGrath and Pitcher 2002; Woodgate 2001, 2006). However, it is important to note that understanding the whole illness experience is important as symptoms cannot be viewed in isolation (Woodgate and Denger 2003). In a study exploring experiences of being in hospital, children and young people with both acute and chronic illnesses described the restrictions that illness symptoms imposed upon them (Edwards 2009). The following quote from one young person with cystic fibrosis (CF) depicts the ways in which the symptoms she experienced impacted upon her life:

> I can't really do anything nowadays because of my CF. Like I can't do any gym stuff anymore, not even when I'm here with the physio because I just get too out of breath. I can't run or anything now. Even just walking to the end of the road makes me out of breath. My appetite's right poor as well. It has been for a while so that affects what I do with my friend or mates. It's no point me going out with them for a meal, not even to MacDonald's because it's a waste of money. I just feel right out of it not eating when they all are. Like they have to think about me all the time and walk slow when I'm there or not walk at all and have to catch a bus. I don't mind too much if it's just [friend] and me because he knows what's it like, but even though my friends know all about CF I still feel as if I'm a pain to them. (Edwards 2009: 145)

Similarly, a child suffering from epilepsy commented that 'it makes me sad when I have headache and tummy ache. And when I have a fit. It tastes horrible' (Edwards 2009: 142).

At present the literature on symptom experience for children and young people is small and primarily focused upon symptoms experienced in cancer. However, it is recognised that fear, fatigue and pain are symptoms experienced by children and young people across a wide range of illnesses.

Fear

Case study 6.6: Harry

Feeling scared

Sometimes Harry is scared of things like going out in the dark at night or the scary monster in Grandad's shed, but now that he is going to hospital he is very frightened. Harry is worried that when they cut his throat open it might not work properly and he won't be able to talk properly (physical fear). He is worried that when he is in hospital he won't know where the toilet is and he might wet his bed like a baby (existential fear) and that when he gets home his friends won't play with him because he can't talk properly (fear of social self). Harry is very scared of going to hospital.

It is widely acknowledged that fear is provoked in pre-school children admitted to hospital due to separation from parents, undergoing nursing procedures and exposure to unfamiliar people (Gozal et al. 2004; Koening et al. 2003; Salmela et al. 2009; Snyder 2004). Fear of the hospital environment itself, equipment, pain (Salmela et al. 2009; Wennstrom and Bergh 2008) injections and needles (Kettwich et al. 2007; Salmela et al. 2009) have also been cited. Coupled with a fear of being in hospital, children and young people may be afraid and anxious regarding their illness and its subsequent treatment. Distress in the form of fear and worries (Hedstrom et al. 2004, 2005) around a threat to self (Anderzen Carlsson et al. 2008), altered appearance (Hedstrom et al. 2005), alienation from friends, medical treatments, dying (Hedstrom et al. 2004) and the unknown (Enskar et al. 1997) have been identified in adolescents with cancer. Fear has been identified in terms of that related to the physical body, the social self, and existential fear (Anderzen Carlsson et al. 2008). Fear relating to the physical body includes: feeling afraid of altered appearance, such as hair loss, weight change and looking different; pain; medical procedures, including surgery, lumbar punctures, injections and needles; bodily complications related to illness and treatment, including intensified smell and taste; death; and fear of staff regarded as unkind. Existential fear meanwhile relates to the unknown, including: uncertainty regarding symptoms and illness; experiencing a loss of control; being admitted to hospital; recurrence of symptoms creating fear of relapse and the need for intensified treatment, evoking a fear both of the treatment itself and of dying. Fear related to the social self includes: a fear of being different; rejection by friends; isolation; and visible signs of illness such as a wheelchair or feeding tube.

It is important for nurses to have an awareness of the factors that can lead to fear in children and young people in order to provide reassurance and to take action to reduce these. Explaining the fears that children and young people may experience to parents can enable families to support them and minimise these anxieties.

Fatigue

While fatigue is associated with many illnesses, including Chronic Fatigue Syndrome (CFS) (Carter and Martin, 2005), its prevalence is most notably studied in children and adolescents with cancer (Hockenberry-Eaton et al. 1998, 1999), with prolonged tiredness frequently cited (CLIC Sargent 2010). Fatigue has been identified as a 'subjective, unpleasant symptom that incorporates total body feelings ranging from tiredness to exhaustion creating an unrelenting overall condition that interferes with individuals' ability to function' (Ream and Richardson 1996: 527). Treatment itself appears to be the main inducer of fatigue (Anderzen Carlsson et al. 2008; Richardson 2004), persisting throughout diagnosis, treatment and the recovery period, with adolescents describing how this continued even between treatments (Gibson et al. 2005). Fatigue can be both physical and mental, with bodily fatigue related to treatment and mental fatigue related to coping with the enormity of the diagnosis (Gibson et al. 2005). The overwhelming nature of fatigue affected adolescents at many levels, with routine hospital visits causing physical and emotional pain and nightmares regarding treatment (Gibson et al. 2005).

When caring for children and young people who are ill and experiencing symptoms it is vital for nurses to be compassionate in the way they are cared for and to acknowledge their symptoms, particularly those such as fatigue that may be invisible to others. Nurses need to be empathetic by listening to children and young people and assessing symptoms accurately in order to provide the best possible treatment, and they have an important role in communicating with parents and families who may be equally anxious and fearful about their child's illness and symptoms.

Pain

Children and young people experience pain not only due to interventions, illness or disability but also as a result of undergoing treatment. As mentioned previously in this chapter, pain has been identified as a significant factor in children's illness and treatment experiences (Kortesluoma and Nikkonen 2006). It is recognised that pain not properly assessed, or addressed by prompt pain relief, can be unpleasant, delay recovery and add to the upset caused by illness, injury or clinical procedures (Department of Health 2004; Health Care Commission 2007). Historically, pain in children has been ineffectively managed (Twycross 2011), with evidence suggesting that it continues to be underestimated, misunderstood and inadequately dealt with (Association of Paediatric Anaesthetists of Great Britain and Ireland 2012; Department of Health 2004). Indeed, research suggests that children continue to experience unrelieved moderate to severe pain post-operatively (Health Care Commission 2007; Taylor et al. 2008), with children themselves perceiving their pain management to be sub-optimal and believing that nurses should take a more active role in communicating with them both about their pain and its management (Johnston et al. 2005; Vincent and Deynes 2004). While guidance on good practice in managing post-operative and procedural pain in children is available (Association of Paediatric Anaesthetists of Great Britain and Ireland 2012), it is noted that gaps in the knowledge of health professionals is a potential barrier in the effective pain management of children (World Health Organization 2012). Indeed, it is argued that the suffering endured by hospitalised children in some low- and middle-income countries is considerable (Forgeron et al. 2006; Jongudomkarn et al. 2006).

It is reported that chronic pain impacts upon the social lives of children in many ways, commonly both affecting sleep and leading to absence from school (Haraldstad et al. 2011). Young people experiencing chronic pain have described this as both a separate entity to, and an intrinsic part of, themselves (Carter et al. 2002a) – constant, difficult to relieve and pervading their lives (Castle et al. 2007). The importance of having their experience of pain acknowledged has been highlighted (Castle et al. 2007). However, although many children and young people want to be involved with health professionals in discussions about their pain (Carter et al. 2002a), many report feeling misunderstood, disbelieved and abandoned (Dell'Api et al. 2007) when they believed that they were not listened to. Children may express their pain through different mediums to adults, for example through drawing (Kortesluoma et al. 2008). With support, children are able to articulate their pain and should be regarded, whenever possible, as the experts about their pain and their insights should be used to optimise pain management (Kortesluoma and Nikkonen, 2004, 2006). Despite this, it has been suggested that a great deal of what we know about their pain experiences has been sought from adults instead of children and young people themselves (Kortesluoma and Nikkonen 2006).

Like illness, children's understanding of pain is affected by many factors such as age, culture, cognitive and linguistic ability, experience and personality. Some children of school age may believe that pain or illness is punishment for being naughty (McGrath and Frager 1996), although other evidence suggests that young children do not link bad behaviour with pain. Adolescents may find it difficult to cope with pain due to their lack of experience of it (Moules and Ramsay 2008). Both fear and anxiety heighten pain (Alder 1991), making those in hospital particularly susceptible to its effects. For children undergoing surgery, post-operative pain has been identified as one of the most intense episodes of pain experienced (Kortesluoma and Nikkonen 2004). However, children view themselves as active agents in pain relief (Franck et al. 2008), using distraction and resting/sleeping in addition to receiving analgesics post-operatively as ways of managing their pain (Polkki et al. 2003; Sng et al. 2013).

It is important to be aware that neonates, infants, critically ill children/young people and those with a complex illness, developmental delay, cognitive impairment or disabilities may be unable to express the pain or symptoms they are experiencing verbally due to their age and/or severity of illness or disability. Children and young people who are unable to report pain may be at an even greater risk of having their pain under-treated (McGrath et al. 1998). Thus, caring for these groups of children and young people can be a particular challenge for nurses. Parents make a unique and important contribution to the management of children's pain through their ability to recognise different behaviour in their child, their ways of expressing pain and the best way to provide comfort (Hong-Gu et al. 2007; Moules and Ramsay 2008). However, it has been argued that parental involvement in their child's pain management is superficial, with parents conveying frustration that their role is passive, limited (Simons et al. 2001) and under-used as a resource by health professionals (Carter et al. 2002b).

For children and young people, the distress at being in hospital and feeling anxious and fearful regarding surgery may all heighten experiences of pain. Hospitalisation together with feeling isolated, afraid and alone can make pain seem all-encompassing. Providing reassurance for children and young people and encouraging them to talk and share their anxieties, alongside optimal pain relief, may help to minimise their distress and pain. Involving parents can also be an effective strategy, particularly in those children and young people who are unable to verbalise their pain.

Case study 6.7: Harry

Waking up after surgery – feeling afraid and in pain

Harry has woken up after the operation feeling very sick. His head feels woozy and his throat is very sore. It hurts to sip water and everyone is telling him to drink more but it makes him feel even more sick than he does already. It hurts a lot and he is worried that everyone will think he is a baby if he cries. He can't understand how this operation has helped his sore throat. He thinks it has made his throat feel even worse. Perhaps if he lies really still and doesn't talk or drink anything the pain will go away.

In summary, children and young people can experience a wide range of illnesses and symptoms, necessitating treatment and procedures. Being ill and undergoing treatment places limitations upon children and young people, provoking fear and anxiety, while the experience of symptoms can cause distress and suffering for children, young people and families. It is important for nurses to acknowledge children's and young people's experiences of illness and symptoms and to assess these accurately in order to ensure the best possible treatment and nursing care.

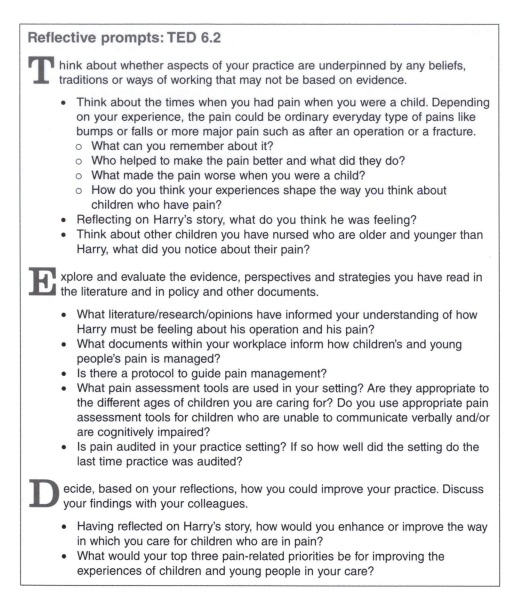

Reflective prompts: TED 6.2

Think about whether aspects of your practice are underpinned by any beliefs, traditions or ways of working that may not be based on evidence.

- Think about the times when you had pain when you were a child. Depending on your experience, the pain could be ordinary everyday type of pains like bumps or falls or more major pain such as after an operation or a fracture.
  o What can you remember about it?
  o Who helped to make the pain better and what did they do?
  o What made the pain worse when you were a child?
  o How do you think your experiences shape the way you think about children who have pain?
- Reflecting on Harry's story, what do you think he was feeling?
- Think about other children you have nursed who are older and younger than Harry, what did you notice about their pain?

Explore and evaluate the evidence, perspectives and strategies you have read in the literature and in policy and other documents.

- What literature/research/opinions have informed your understanding of how Harry must be feeling about his operation and his pain?
- What documents within your workplace inform how children's and young people's pain is managed?
- Is there a protocol to guide pain management?
- What pain assessment tools are used in your setting? Are they appropriate to the different ages of children you are caring for? Do you use appropriate pain assessment tools for children who are unable to communicate verbally and/or are cognitively impaired?
- Is pain audited in your practice setting? If so how well did the setting do the last time practice was audited?

Decide, based on your reflections, how you could improve your practice. Discuss your findings with your colleagues.

- Having reflected on Harry's story, how would you enhance or improve the way in which you care for children who are in pain?
- What would your top three pain-related priorities be for improving the experiences of children and young people in your care?

Conclusion

This chapter has considered children's and young people's experiences of illness and symptoms and the ways in which these impact upon children and young people and their families. Children and young people are concerned about different aspects of being ill to adults and their understanding of illness is dependent upon factors such as their age, experience, personality and cognitive ability. Being ill and undergoing treatment impacts upon children's and young peoples' lives and can feel all-encompassing, particularly for those with long-term illnesses.

References

Admi, H. (1996) 'Growing up with a chronic health condition: a model of an ordinary life-style', *Qualitative Health Research*, 6(2): 163–183.

Alder, S. (1991) 'Taking children at their word: pain control in paediatrics', *Professional Nurse*, 5(8): 398–402.

Anderzen Carlsson, A., Kihlgren, A. and Sorlie, V. (2008) 'Embodied suffering: experiences of fear in adolescent girls with cancer', *Journal of Child Health Care*, 12(2): 129–143.

Association of Paediatric Anaesthetists of Great Britain and Ireland (2012) 'Good practice in postoperative and procedural pain management', *Pediatric Anesthesia*, 22: Supplement 1: 1–79.

Archard, R. (1993) *Children: Rights and Childhood*. London: Routledge.

Atkin, K. and Ahmad, W.I.U. (2001) 'Living a 'normal' life: young people coping with thalas-saemia major or sickle cell disorder', *Social Science & Medicine*, 53(5): 615–626.

Battrick, C. and Glasper, E.A. (2004) 'The views of children and their families on being in hospital', *British Journal of Nursing*, 13(6): 328–336.

Beale, H. (2002) 'Respite care for technology-dependent children and their families', *Paediatric Nursing*, 14(7): 18–19.

Berman, H. (2003) 'Getting critical with children: empowering approaches with a disempow-ered group', *Advanced in Nursing Science*, 26(2): 102–113.

Bjorkman, B., Almqvist, L., Sigstedt, B. and Enskar, K. (2012) 'Children's experience of going through an acute radiographic examination', *Radiography*, 18(2): 84–89.

Bluebond-Langner, M. (1978) *The Private Worlds of Dying Children*. Princeton: Princeton University Press.

Board, R.M. (2005) 'School-age children's perceptions of their PICU hospitalization', *Pediatric Nursing*, 31(3): 166–175.

Board, R.M. and Ryan-Wenger, N. (2002) 'Long-term effects of PICU hospitalization on families with young children', *Heart & Lung: The Journal of Acute and Critical Care* 31(1): 53–66.

Bsiri-Moghaddam, K., Bsiri-Moghaddam, M., Sadeghmoghaddam, L. and Ahmadi, F. (2011) 'The concept of hospitalization of children from the view point of parent and children', *Iran Journal of Pediatrics*, 21(2): 201–208.

Bricher, G. (2000) 'Children in the hospital: issues of power and vulnerability', *Pediatric Nursing*, 26(3): 277–282.

Buckley, A. and Savage, E. (2010) 'Preoperative information needs of children undergoing tonsillectomy', *Journal of Clinical Nursing*, 19(19–20): 2879–2887.

Bunn, M. (2010) *No Secrets. Helping Families and Carers Talk to Children about Life-Limiting Illness*. Malawi: Umodzi.

Carnevale, F.A., Alexander, E., Davis, M., Rennick, J.E. and Troini, R. (2006) 'Daily living with distress and enrichment: the moral experience of families with ventilator assisted children at home', *Pediatrics*, 117(1): e48–e60.

Carney, T., Murphy, S., McClure, J., Bishop, E., Kerr, C., Parker, J., Scott, F., Shields, C. and Wilson, L. (2003) 'Children's views of hospitalization: an exploratory study of data collec-tion', *Journal of Child Health Care*, 7(1): 27–40.

Carter, B. (2005) '"They've got to be as good as mum and dad": Children with complex needs and their siblings' perceptions of a Diana community nursing service', *Clinical Effectiveness in Nursing*, 9(1–2): 49–61.

Carter, B. (2014) '"Just kids playing sport (in a chair)'": experiences of children, fami-lies and stakeholders attending a wheelchair sports club, *Disability and Sport*, doi: 101080/09687599.2014.880329.

Carter, B. and Martin, L. (2005) *Persistence and Resistance in Worlds made Uncertain by CFS/ ME*. Report Submitted to *AYME*. University of Central Lancashire.

Carter, B., Lambrenos, K. and Thursfield, J. (2002a) 'A pain workshop: an approach to eliciting the views of young people with chronic pain', *Journal of Clinical Nursing*, 11(6): 753–762.

Carter, B., McArthur, E. and Cunliffe, M. (2002b) 'Dealing with uncertainty: parental assessment of pain in their children with profound special needs', *Journal of Advanced Nursing*, 38(5): 449–457.

Carter, B., Edwards, M. and Hunt, A. (2013) '"Being a presence": the ways in which family support workers encompass, embrace, befriend, accompany and endure with families of life-limited children', *Journal of Child Health Care*, Online First, doi: 10.1177/1367493513516391.

Castle, K., Imms, C. and Howie, L. (2007) 'Being in pain: a phenomenological study of young people with cerebral palsy', *Developmental Medicine and Child Neurology*, 49(6): 445–449.

Chesney, M., Lindeke, L., Johnson, L., Jukkala, A. and Lynch, S. (2005) 'Comparison of child and parent satisfaction ratings of ambulatory pediatric subspeciality care', *Journal of Pediatric Health Care*, 19(4): 221–229.

Christian, B.J. and D'Auria, J.P. (1997) 'The child's eye: memories of growing up with cystic fibrosis', *Journal of Pediatric Nursing*, 12(1): 3–12.

Clarke-Steffen, L. (1993) 'Waiting and not knowing: the diagnosis of cancer in a child', *Journal of Pediatric Oncology Nursing*, 10(4): 146–153.

CLIC Sargent (2010) *The Impact of Cancer on a Child's World: The Views of Children Aged 7 to 13 Living With and Beyond Cancer*. London: CLIC Sargent.

CLIC Sargent (2011) *Counting the Costs of Cancer: The Financial Impact of Cancer on Children, Young People and their Families*. London: CLIC Sargent.

Cohen, M.H. (1993) 'The unknown and the unknowable – managing sustained uncertainty', *Western Journal of Nursing Research*, 15(1): 77–96.

Comaroff, J. and Maguire, P. (1981) 'Ambiguity and the search for meaning: childhood leukaemia in the modern clinical context', *Social Science & Medicine*, 15(2): 115–123.

Coyne, I. (2003) *A grounded theory of disrupted lives: children, parents and nurses in the children's ward*. Unpublished PhD thesis, University of London.

Coyne, I. (2006) 'Consultation with children in hospital: children, parents' and nurses' perspectives', *Journal of Clinical Nursing*, 15(1): 61–71.

Crisp, J., Ungerer, J. and Goodnow, J. (1996) 'The impact of experience on children's understanding of illness', *Journal of Pediatric Psychology*, 21(1): 57–72.

Darvill, J., Harrington, A. and Donovan, J. (2009) 'Caring for ventilated children at home: the child's perspective', *Neonatal, Paediatric and Child Health Nursing*, 12(3): 9–13.

Dell'Api, M., Rennick, J.E. and Rosmus, C. (2007) 'Childhood chronic pain and health care professional interactions: shaping the chronic pain experiences of children', *Journal of Child Health Care*, 11(4): 269–286.

Department of Health (2004) *National Standards Framework for Children, Young People and Maternity Services: Core Standards*. London: Department of Health.

Department of Health (2011) *NHS at Home: Community Children's Nursing Services*. London: Department of Health.

Docherty, S. and Sandelowski, M. (1999) 'Focus on qualitative methods: interviewing children', *Research in Nursing and Health*, 22(2): 177–185.

Drendell, A.L., Lyon, R., Bergholte, J. and Kim, M.K. (2006) 'Outpatient pediatric pain management practices for fractures', *Pediatric Emergency Care*, 22(2): 94–99.

Edwards, M.E.B. (2009) *Children's and young people's experiences of being in hospital: disruption, uncertainty, powerlessness and restoring equilibrium*. Unpublished PhD thesis, University of Central Lancashire.

Eiser, C. (1990) *Chronic Childhood Disease*. Cambridge: Cambridge University Press.

Eklund, P.G. and Sivberg, B. (2003) 'Adolescents' lived experience of epilepsy', *Journal of Neuroscience Nursing*, 35(1): 40–49.

Enskar, K., Carlsson, M., Golsater, M. and Hamrin, E. (1997) 'Symptom distress and life situation in adolescents with cancer', *Cancer Nursing*, 20(1): 23–33.

Fletcher, T., Glasper, A., Prudhoe, G., Battrick, C., Coles, L., Weaver, K. and Ireland, L. (2011) 'Building the future: children's views on nurses and hospital care', *British Journal of Nursing*, 20(1): 39–45.

Ford, K. (2011) '"I didn't really like it, but it sounded exciting": admission to hospital for surgery from the perspectives of children', *Journal of Child Health Care*, 15(4): 250–260.

Ford, K., Courtney-Pratt, H. and FitzGerald, M. (2012) 'Post-discharge experiences of children and their families following children's surgery', *Journal of Child Health Care*, 16(4): 320–330.

Forinder, U. (2004) 'Bone marrow transplantation from a parental perspective', *Journal of Child Health Care*, 8(2): 134–148.

Forinder, U. and Posse, E. (2008) '"A life on hold": adolescents' experiences of stem cell transplantation in a long-term perspective', *Journal of Child Health Care*, 12(4): 301–313.

Forgeron, P.A., Finley, G.A. and Arnaout, M. (2006) 'Pediatric pain prevalence and parents' attitudes at a cancer hospital in Jordan', *Journal of Pain and Symptom Management*, 31(5):438–446.

Forsner, M., Jansson, L. and Sorlie, V. (2005a) 'The experience of being ill as narrated by hospitalised children aged 7–10 years with short-term illness', *Journal of Child Health Care*, 9(2): 153–165.

Forsner, M., Jansson, L. and Sorlie, V. (2005b) 'Being ill as narrated by children aged 11–18 years', *Journal of Child Health Care*, 9(4): 314–323.

Fortier, M.A., Chorney, J.M., Rony, R.Y., Perret-Karimi, D., Rinehart, J.B. Camilon, F.S. and Kain, Z.N. (2009) 'Children's desire for perioperative information', *Anesthesia and Analgesia*, 109(4): 1085–1090.

Franck, L.S., Sheikh, A. and Oulton, K. (2008) 'What helps when it hurts: children's views on pain relief', *Child: Care, Health & Development*, 34(4): 430–438.

Gibson, F., Mulhall, A.B., Edwards, J.L., Ream, E. and Sepion, B.J. (2005) 'A phenomenologic study of fatigue in adolescents receiving treatment for cancer', *Oncology Nursing Forum*, 32(3): 651–660.

Glendinning, C., Kirk, S., Guiffridda, A. and Lawton, D. (1999) *The Community-based Care of Technology Dependent Children in the UK: Definitions, Numbers and Costs*, National Primary Care Research and Development Centre. Manchester: University of Manchester.

Gozal, D., Drengren, B., Levin, P., Kadari, A. and Gozal, Y. (2004) 'A pediatric sedation/anesthesia program with dedicated care by anaesthesiologists and nurses for procedures outside the operating room', *Journal of Pediatrics*, 145(1): 47–52.

Haraldstad, K., Sørum, R., Eide, H., Natvig, G.K. and Helseth, S. (2011) 'Pain in children and adolescents: prevalence, impact on daily life and parents' perception, a school survey', *Scandinavian Journal of Caring Sciences*, 25(1): 27–36.

Health Care Commission (2007) *Improving Services for Children in Hospital*. London: Health Care Commission.

Hedstrom, M., Haglund, K., Skolin, I. and von Essen, L. (2003) 'Distressing events for children and adolescents with cancer: child, parent and nurse perceptions', *Journal of Pediatric Oncology Nursing*, 20(3): 120–132.

Hedstrom, M., Ljungman, G. and von Essen, L. (2005) 'Perceptions of distress among adolescents recently diagnosed with cancer', *Journal of Pediatric Hematology/Oncology*, 27(1): 6–17.

Hedstrom, M., Skolin, I. and von Essen, L. (2004) 'Distressing and positive experiences and important aspects of care for adolescents treated for cancer. Adolescent and nurse perceptions', *European Journal of Oncology Nursing*, 8(1): 6–17.

Hewitt-Taylor, J. (2008) *Children with Complex and Continuing Health Needs: The Experiences of Children, Families and Care Staff*. London: Jessica Kingsley Publishers.

Hockenberry-Eaton, M., Hinds, P.S., Alcoser, P., O'Neill, J.B., Euell, K. and Howard, V. (1998) 'Fatigue in children and adolescents with cancer', *Journal of Pediatric Oncology Nursing*, 15(3): 172–182.

Hockenberry-Eaton, M., Hinds, P., O'Neill, J.B., Alcoser, P., Bottomley, S. and Kline, N.E. (1999) 'Developing a conceptual model for fatigue in children', *European Journal of Oncology Nursing*, 3(1): 5–11.

Hogan, D. (2006) 'Researching "the child" in developmental psychology', in S. Greene and D. Hogan (eds) *Researching Children's Experience*. London: Sage.

Hong-Gu, H., Vehvilainen-Julkunen, K., Polkki, T. and Pietila, A.M. (2007) 'Children's perceptions on the implementation of methods for their postoperative pain alleviation: an interview study', *International Journal of Nursing Practice*, 13(2): 89–99.

Horner, S.D. (1999) 'Asthma self care: just another piece of school work', *Pediatric Nursing*, 25(597): 600–604.

International Children's Palliative Care Network (ICPCN) (2012) 'September is childhood cancer awareness month', *News Bulletin*, 3 September. Available at: www.icpcn.org.uk

James, A., Jenks, C. and Prout, A. (2001) 'The presociological child', in A. James, C. Jenks and A. Prout (eds) *Theorizing Childhood*. Cambridge: Polity Press.

Jessop, D.J. and Stein, R.E.K. (1985) 'Uncertainty and its relationship to the psychological and social correlates of chronic illness in children', *Social Science & Medicine*, 20(10): 993–999.

Johnston, C.C., Gagnon, A.J., Pepler, C.J. and Bourgault, P. (2005) 'Pain in the emergency department with one-week follow-up of pain resolution', *Pain Research and Management*, 10(2): 67–70.

Jongudomkarn, D., Aungsupakorn, N. and Camfield, L. (2006) 'The meanings of pain: a qualitative study of the perspectives of children living with pain in north-eastern Thailand', *Nursing and Health Sciences*, 8(3): 156–163.

Jones, S.M., Fiser, D.H. and Livingston, R.L. (1992) 'Behavioural changes in pediatric intensive care units', *American Journal of Disabled Children*, 146(3): 375–379.

Kennedy, I. (2001) *The Report of the Public Inquiry into Children's Heart Surgery at the Bristol Royal Infirmary 1984–1995: Learning from Bristol*. London: The Stationery Office.

Kettwich, S., Sibbitt, W., Brandt, J., Johnson, C., Wong, C. and Bankhurst, A. (2007) 'Needle phobia and stress reducing medical devices in pediatric and adult chemotherapy patients', *Journal of Pediatric Oncology Nursing*, 24(1): 20–28.

Kim, Y. and Morrow, G. (2003) 'Changes in family relationships affect the development of chemotherapy-related nausea symptoms', *Journal of Supportive Care in Cancer*, 11(3): 171–177.

Kirk, S. (1999) 'Caring for children with specialized health care needs in the community: the challenges for primary care', *Health & Social Care in the Community*, 7(5): 350–357.

Kirk, S., Glendinning, C. and Callery, P. (2005) 'The experience of being the parent of a technology-dependent child', *Journal of Advanced Nursing*, 51(5): 456–464.

Koening, K., Chesla, C. and Kennedy, C. (2003) 'Parents' perspectives of asthma crisis hospital management in infants and toddlers: an interpretive view through the lens of attachment theory', *Journal of Pediatric Nursing*, 18(4): 233–242.

Kortesluoma, R.L. and Nikkonen, M. (2004) '"I had this horrible pain": the sources and causes of pain experiences in 4- to 11-year-old hospitalized children', *Journal of Child Health Care*, 8(3): 210–231.

Kortesluoma, R.L. and Nikkonen, M. (2006) '"The most disgusting ever": children's pain descriptions and views of the purpose of pain', *Journal of Child Health Care*, 10(3): 213–227.

Kortesluoma, R.L., Punamaki, R.L. and Nikkonen, M. (2008) 'Hospitalized children drawing their pain: the contents and emotional characteristics of pain drawings', *Journal of Child Health Care*, 12(4): 284–300.

Lansdown, G. (2009) *See Me, Hear Me: A Guide to Using the UN Convention on the Rights of Persons with Disabilities to Promote the Rights of Children.* London: Save the Children.

LeRoy, S., Elixson, M., O'Brien, P., Tong, E., Turpin, S. and Uzark, K. (2003) 'Recommendations for preparing children and adolescents for invasive cardiac procedures', *Circulation. American Heart Association Scientific Statement*, 108: 2550–2564.

Lindsay Waters, A. (2008) 'An ethnography of a children's renal unit: experiences of children and young people with long-term renal illness', *Journal of Clinical Nursing*, 17(23): 3103–3114.

Lumeng, J.C., Warschausky, S.A., Nelson, V.S. and Augenstein, K. (2001) 'The quality of life of ventilator-assisted children', *Pediatric Rehabilitation* 4 (1): 21–27.

Lyons, S., Corneille, D., Coker, P. and Ellis, C. (2009) 'A miracle in the outfield: the benefits of participation in organized baseball leagues for children with mental and physical disabilities', *Therapeutic Recreation Journal*, 43(3): 41–48.

MacDonald, H. and Callery, P. (2007) 'Parenting children requiring complex care: a journey through time', *Child Care, Health and Development*, 34(2): 207–213.

Marshall, M. (2010) 'Living with diabetes: normal but different, different but normal', *Endocrine Abstracts*, 24: 526.

Marshall, M., Carter, B. and Brotherton, A. (2009) 'Living with type 1 diabetes: perceptions of children and their parents', *Journal of Clinical* Nursing, 18(12): 1703–1710.

Massie, R. and Massie, S. (1975) *Journey.* New York: Alfred A. Knopf.

McCallin, A., Dickinson, A.R. and Weston, K. (2007) *Family Support for Children with Complex Disabilities: Time for Action.* Auckland: Waitemata District Health Board, AUT University.

McGrath, P. and Pitcher, L. (2002) '"Enough is enough": qualitative findings on the impact of dexamethasone during reinduction/consolidation for paediatric acute lymphoblastic leukaemia', *Journal of Supportive Care in Cancer*, 10(2): 146–155.

McGrath, P.J. and Frager, G. (1996) 'Psychological barriers to optimal pain management in infants and children', *Clinical Journal of Pain*, 12(2): 135–141.

McGrath, P.J., Finley, G.A., Johnston, C.C., Stevens, B.J., von Baeyer, C.L. and Craig, K.D. (1998) 'Behaviours caregivers use to determine pain in non-verbal, cognitively impaired individuals', *Developmental Medicine & Child Neurology*, 40(5): 340–343.

Meadows, S. (1993) *The Child as a Thinker: The Development and Acquisition of Cognition in Childhood.* London: Routledge.

Milligan, C. and Whiles, J. (2010) 'Landscapes of care', *Progress in Human Geography*, 34(6): 736–754.

Moore, A., Anderson, C., Carter, B. and Coad, J. (2010) 'Appropriated landscapes: the intrusion of technology and equipment into the homes and lives of families with a child with complex needs', *Journal of Child Health Care*, 14(1): 3–5.

Moules, T. and Ramsay, J. (2008) *The Textbook of Children's and Young People's Nursing*, 2nd edn. Oxford: Blackwell Publishing.

Nilsson, S., Finnstrom, B., Kokinsky, E. and Enskar, K. (2009) 'The use of virtual reality for needle-related procedural pain and distress in children and adolescents in a paediatric oncology unit', *European Journal of Oncology Nursing*, 13(2): 102–109.

Noyes, J. (1999) 'The impact of knowing your child is critically ill: a qualitative study of mothers' experiences', *Journal of Advanced Nursing*, 29(2): 427–435.

Noyes, J. (2000) 'Enabling young ventilator-dependent people to express their views and experiences of their care in hospital', *Journal of Advanced Nursing*, 31(5): 1206–1215.

Ortiz, M.I., Lopez-Zarco, M. and Arreola-Bautista, E.J. (2012) 'Procedural pain and anxiety in paediatric patients in a Mexican emergency department', *Journal of Advanced Nursing*, 68(12): 2700–2709.

Pelander, T. and Leino-Kilpi, H. (2010) 'Children's best and worst experiences during hospitalisation', *Scandinavian Journal of Caring Sciences*, 24(4): 726–733.

Place, B. (2000) 'Constructing the bodies of critically ill children: an ethnography of intensive care', in A. Prout (ed.) *The Body, Childhood and Society*. London: Macmillan.

Polkki, T., Pietila, A. and Vehvilainen-Julkunen, K. (2003) 'Hospitalized children's descriptions of their experiences with postsurgical pain relieving methods', *International Journal of Nursing Studies*, 40(1): 33–44.

Ream, E. and Richardson, A. (1996) 'Fatigue: a concept analysis', *International Journal of Nursing Studies*, 33(5): 519–529.

Rennick, J.E., Morin, L., Kim, D., Johnston, C.C., Dougherty, G. and Platt, R. (2004) 'Identifyng children at high risk for psychological sequelae after pediatric intensive care unit hospitalization', *Pediatric Critical Care Medicine*, 5(4): 358–363.

Richardson, A. (2004) 'A critical appraisal of the factors associated with fatigue', in J. Armes, M. Krishnasamy and I. Higginson (eds) *Fatigue in Cancer*. Oxford: Oxford University Press.

Rhee, H., Wenzel, J. and Stevens, R.H. (2007) 'Adolescents' psychosocial experiences living with asthma: a focus group study', *Journal of Pediatric Health Care*, 21(2): 99–107.

Rydstrom, I., Dalheim Englund, A.C. and Sandman, P.O. (1999) 'Being a child with asthma', *Pediatric Nursing*, 25(6): 589–596.

Royal College of Nursing (RCN) (2011) *Health Care Standards in Caring for Neonates, Children and Young People*. London: Royal College of Nursing.

Salmela, M., Aronen, E.T. and Salanterä, S. (2010) 'The experience of hospital-related fears of 4- to 6-year-old children', *Child: Care, Health & Development*, 37(5): 719–726.

Salmela, M., Salanterä, S. and Aronen, E.T. (2009) 'Child-reported hospital fears of 4 to 6-year-old children', *Pediatric Nursing*, 35(5): 269–276.

Save the Children (1989) *Hospital: A Deprived Environment for Children?* London: Save the Children.

Sigelman, C., Maddock, A., Epstein, J. and Carpenter, W. (1993) 'Age differences in understandings of disease causality – Aids, colds and cancer', *Child Development*, 64(1): 272–284.

Simons, J., Franck, L. and Robertson, E. (2001) 'Parent involvement in children's pain care: views of parents and nurses', *Journal of Advanced Nursing*, 36(4): 591–599.

Smith, L. and Callery, P. (2005) 'Children's accounts of their pre-operative information needs', *Journal of Clinical Nursing*, 14(2): 230–238.

Snyder, B. (2004) 'Preventing treatment interference: nurses' and parents' intervention strategies', *Paediatric Nursing*, 30(1): 31–40.

Sng, Q.W., Taylor, B., Liam, J.L., Klainin-Yobas, P., Wang, W. and He, H.G. (2013) 'Postoperative pain management experiences among school-aged children: a qualitative study', *Journal of Clinical Nursing*, 22(7–8): 958–968.

Sourkes, B., Frankel, L. and Brown, M. (2005) 'Food, toys and love: pediatric palliative care', *Current Problems in Pediatric and Adolescent Health Care*, 35(9): 350–386.

Southall, D., Burr, A., Smith, R., Bull, D., Williams, A. and Nicholson, S. (2000) 'The child friendly healthcare initiative (CFHI): healthcare provision in accordance with the UN Convention on the Rights of the Child', *Pediatrics*, 106(5): 1054–1064.

Stalker, K., Carpenter, J., Phillips, R., Connors, C., MacDonald, C., Eyre, J., Noyes, J., Chaplin, S. and Place, M. (2003) *Care and Treatment? Supporting Children with Complex Needs in Healthcare Settings*. Brighton: Pavilion Publishing.

Steele, R. (2005) 'Strategies used by families to navigate unchartered territory when a child is dying', *Journal of Palliative Care*, 21(2): 103–110.

Stefanatou, A. (2008) 'Use of drawings in children with pervasive developmental disorder during hospitalization: a developmental perspective', *Journal of Child Health Care*, 12(4): 268–283.

Sterken, D. (1996) 'Uncertainty and coping in fathers of children with cancer', *Journal of Pediatric Oncology Nursing*, 13(2): 81–88.

Stewart, J.L. (2003) '"Getting used to it": children finding the ordinary and routine in the uncertain context of cancer', *Qualitative Health Research*, 13(3): 394–407.

Taylor, R.M., Gibson, F. and Franck, L.S. (2008) 'The experience of living with a chronic illness during adolescence: a critical review of the literature', *Journal of Clinical Nursing*, 17(23): 3083–3091.

Teixeira, E.M.D. and de Figueiredo, M.C.B. (2009) 'The child's preoperative experience in a planned surgery' (Portugese), *Revista Cientifica da Unidade de Investigacao em Ciencias da Saude: Dominio de Enfermagem (REFERENCIA)*, 9: 7–14.

The Children's Society (2011) *4 in Every 10 Disabled Children Living in Poverty*. London: The Children's Society.

The Paediatric Society of New Zealand (2002) *Consultation Draft. New Zealand Standards for the Wellbeing of Children and Adolescents Receiving Healthcare*. The Paediatric Society of New Zealand.

Twycross, A. (2011) 'Principles of pain management and entitlement to pain relief', in R. Davies and A. Davies (eds) *Children and Young People's Nursing: Principles for Practice*. London: Hodder & Stoughton.

United Nations (2007) *Millennium Development Goals Indicators Database*. New York: United Nations.

Vincent, C.V.H. and Deynes, M.J. (2004) 'Relieving children's pain: nurses' abilities and analgesic administration practices', *Journal of Pediatric Nursing*, 19(1): 40–50.

Wennstrom, L. and Bergh, I. (2008) 'Bodily and verbal expressions of postoperative symptoms in 3- to 6-year old boys', *Journal of Pediatric Nursing*, 23(1): 65–76.

Wilson, M.E., Megel, M.E., Enenbach, L. and Carlson, K.L. (2010) 'The voices of children: stories about hospitalization', *Journal of Pediatric Health Care*, 24(2): 95–102.

Wise, B.V. (2002) 'In their own words: the lived experience of pediatric liver transplantation', *Qualitative Health Research*, 12(1): 74–90.

Wong, M.Y.F. and Chan, S.W.C. (2006) 'The qualitative experience of Chinese parents with children diagnosed of cancer', *Journal of Clinical Nursing*, 15(6): 710–717.

Woodhead, M. (1997) 'Psychology and the cultural construction of children's needs', in A. James and A. Prout (eds) *Constructing and Reconstructing Childhood*. London: Falmer Press.

Woodgate, R.L. (2001) *Symptom experiences in the illness trajectory of children with cancer and their families*. PhD thesis, University of Manitoba.

Woodgate, R.L. (2006) 'Life is never the same: childhood cancer narratives', *European Journal of Cancer Care*, 15(1): 8–18.

Woodgate, R. and Denger, L. (2003) '"Nothing is carved in stone!" Uncertainty in children with cancer and their families', *European Journal of Oncology Nursing*, 6(4): 191–202.

World Health Organization (2012) *WHO Guidelines on the Pharmacological Treatment of Persisting Pain in Children with Medical Illnesses*. Geneva: WHO.

Yoos, H.L. and McMullen, A. (1996) 'Illness narratives of children with asthma', *Pediatric Nursing*, 22(4): 285–290.

Young, B., Dixon-Woods, M., Windridge, K.C. and Heney, D. (2002) 'Parenting in crisis: Conceptualizing mothers of children with cancer', *Social Science & Medicine*, 55(10): 1835–1847.

Chapter 7

Examining Practice: Improving the Care of Children and Young People

Key points

- The notion of 'best practice' is frequently espoused by nurses caring for children and families; however, understanding of what this actually means is influenced by the culture and context in which it is used.
- Best practice can be presented from the perspective of research, quality and risk management, professional standards and that of the children and families themselves.
- There are a number of ways in which best practice is evaluated and these include: evaluative research, internal audit, complaint or error reporting and benchmarking.
- Developing and changing practice requires a carefully planned change process which is considerate of the climate for practice change and the responses of those affected by or participating in the practice development.
- Health care organisations and nursing services which embrace Evidence Based Practice (EBP), innovation and practice have demonstrated improved outcomes in relation to nursing practice and patient outcomes.
- A strong culture of innovation and practice development is reliant on: effective partnerships between researchers and clinicians, health services which value and demand quality and innovation, effective engagement with children and families, strong nursing leadership and the willingness of nurses to engage in practice development.

Key theories and concepts explored in this chapter are best practice, quality, change management and practice development.

Case study 7.1: Beth

Setting the scene

Beth was the quality leader at the children's hospital. A government target had been set to improve the oral health of the country's children and in support of this the hospital

(Continued)

(Continued)

nursing service decided to review oral care practices. While Beth suspected that oral care was often overlooked in hospital she had difficulty convincing the nurses that this practice required review. Nurses in the Oncology Unit said that their practice did not need reviewing as they already had in place an oral care protocol for children on chemotherapy. PICU nurses had also recently introduced a new clinical guideline and the nurses in the emergency and acute care areas did not see the necessity because of the short stays of children in their area. However, Beth was determined that the nursing service should play its part in meeting the government target. Little was known about how nurses in the hospital assessed, maintained and promoted children's oral health. Although the hospital did purchase an array of oral health care products, if a family did not bring a toothbrush or toothpaste in with them it was almost impossible to find one in the hospital supply cupboard. Beth's suspicions in regard to practice were confirmed when a survey revealed that only 63% of the nurses undertook oral health care assessments, with only 26% being confident that oral health care was regularly promoted and carried out in their area. Nurses who gave oral care were most likely to use products (Chlorhexidine, sterile water, mouth swabs) and practices unsupported by best evidence. Nurses did not support the enrolment of children in the national dental services. The survey revealed that nurses knew little about the process of enrolment and when asked gave inaccurate information in regard to age of enrolment. In response to this Beth and her team set about developing clinical guidelines and assessment tools which were accompanied by a hospital-wide nursing education programme. Management and local businesses supported the hospital's oral health campaign which ran parallel to the wider national campaign. Six months post implementation Beth optimistically awaited the survey results confident that practice had improved. However, this optimism soon dissipated when the survey results revealed that little had changed. The majority of nurses still did not carry out regular oral health assessments and a wide array of products which were unsupported by best evidence continued to be used. Despite the increased availability of educational resources only a minority of nurses were actively promoting oral health care. While there was increased awareness of what they 'should' do most nurses continued to do what they had always done.

Introduction

Nurses who care for children and young people are increasingly called to ensure that care delivered reflects 'best practice' and that it is developed and improved to ensure quality of care and good health outcomes for children and families. To do this nurses are called to review and challenge 'taken for granted' practices and asked to consider new and innovative ways of providing nursing care. This chapter will critically review the notion of 'best practice' and consider the factors which facilitate or challenge the development of quality practice with children and their families.

What is best practice?

Over recent decades the concept of quality health care has come to the fore and inherent within this is the notion of ensuring that nurses and other health professionals deliver care which reflects 'best practice'. It is no longer acceptable for a nurse to deliver care based on what she/he alone feels is best for the child and family, based on experiential knowledge or preference. Nurses must now ensure that the care they deliver is supported by the best available evidence, taking into account contextual considerations and the particular needs of the child and their family. Nursing practice outside of such parameters is now open to challenge from not only legal, regulatory and professional groups but also from colleagues, employees and increasingly from consumer groups and children and families.

So what is best practice? A review of the literature would suggest that there are four prominent views on best practice: firstly the scientific view reflected within the Evidence Based Nursing (EBN) literature; secondly the government or organisational view reflected in policy and quality management systems; thirdly the professional view reflected in standards and competencies; and fourthly a consumer view often reflected through the media or consumer advocacy groups.

The scientific view: evidence based nursing

The most dominant view of best practice within health care is that which has arisen from the Evidence Based Practice (EBP) movement which views best practice as that which is based on the best available evidence. Following its origins in Evidence Based Medicine (EBM), EBP is described as practice which is based on valid scientific research and the strength of evidence is graded according to levels of evidence using EBM frameworks, with Randomised Control Trials (RCT) being considered the most reliable (Scott and McSherry 2009) (see Table 7.1).

Difficulties in identifying sufficient evidence using such narrow categories and the growing recognition that such a framework fails to account for contextual issues and the nature of nursing have led to broader definitions being put forward, such as those by Pearson et al. (2005) who view EBP as: 'clinical decision-making that considers the best available evidence; the context in which care is delivered; client preference; and the professional judgement of the health professional' (p. 209). While more inclusive than previous definitions, it is still determined by the support of 'legitimate evidence' (Pearson et al. 2005). Best practice from this perspective is that in which the nurse delivers care and makes clinical decisions with the child and family based on the best available evidence which has been critically reviewed and considered in relation to the patient and the context in which they are being cared for.

Case study 7.2: Beth

Finding the evidence

Beth and her team initially turned to the scientific evidence for guidance in regard to the development of the assessment tool and practice guidelines. However, despite searching a number of databases and having the assistance of the medical librarian, they were unable to locate any Level 1 or 2 studies using FAME (see Table 7.1)and found that the majority of the literature was graded as Level 4. While the scientific perspective informed the project it did not give clear direction to the team.

Table 7.1 The Joanne Briggs Institute (JBI) Levels of Evidence FAME

Levels of Evidence	Feasibility F(1–4)	Appropriateness A(1–4)	Meaningfulness M(1–4)	Effectiveness E(1–4)	Economic Evidence
1	Metasynthesis of research with unequivocal synthesised findings	Metasynthesis of research with unequivocal synthesised findings	Metasynthesis of research with unequivocal synthesised findings	Meta-analysis(with homogeneity) of experimental studies (e.g. RCT with concealed randomisation) OR One or more large experimental studies with narrow confidence intervals	Metasynthesis (with homogeneity) of evaluations of important alternative interventions comparing all clinically relevant outcomes against appropriate cost measurement, and including a clinically sensible sensitivity analysis
2	Metasynthesis of research with credible synthesised findings	Metasynthesis of research with credible synthesised findings	Metasynthesis of research with credible synthesised findings	One or more smaller RCTs with wider confidence intervals OR Quasi-experimental studies(without randomisation)	Evaluations of important alternative interventions comparing all clinically relevant outcomes against appropriate cost measurement, and including a clinically sensible sensitivity analysis
3	a. Metasynthesis of text/opinion with credible synthesised findings b. One or more single research studies of high quality	a. Metasynthesis of text/opinion with credible synthesised findings b. One or more single research studies of high quality	a. Metasynthesis of text/opinion with credible synthesised findings b. One or more single research studies of high quality	a. Cohort studies (with control group) b. Case-controlled c. Observational studies(without control group)	Evaluations of important alternative interventions comparing a limited number of appropriate cost measurement, without a clinically sensible sensitivity analysis
4	Expert opinion	Expert opinion	Expert opinion	Expert opinion, or physiology bench research, or consensus	Expert opinion, or based on economic theory

While the nursing literature continues to debate the fit of EBP within the nursing context (Scott and McSherry 2009; Wall 2008), it is clear that EBP will be a dominant influence in defining best practice within nursing and health care services.

The government and organisational view

The second view of best practice is that reflected by government and organisations which fund and deliver health services to children and families. This view of best practice is usually linked to regulation, resource allocation and quality management, including key performance indicators and targets. While in most instances there will be a direct link to best evidence or guidelines developed using EBN principles, sometimes tensions arise when the practice supported by EBN conflicts with components of best practice as described by government or health care organisations. Tensions often relate to recommended drugs or treatments and organisational quality targets which do not necessarily integrate well. While the best practice literature supports close alignment between the evidence, government, and organisational factors in the development of best practice guidelines (Marchionni and Ritchie 2008b), this is not always the case.

Case study 7.3: Beth

Best practice determined by targets

In New Zealand, where Beth practices, government organisations describe best oral care practices as those where children and young people are enrolled in a dental health service, have regular examinations of their teeth and gums by health professionals, and parents are appropriately referred on to specialist dental services. For the oral health strategy, specific resources were allocated and targets set against which best practice could be measured. However, for Beth, meeting these predetermined targets was not always going to be easy because of another government target related to best practice in the emergency department which required that children and families stay less than six hours in the Emergency Department. This often precluded the nursing staff from addressing opportunistic oral health assessments and referrals as recommended in the best practice guidelines. This may have contributed to the emergency nurses' reluctance to engage with the project.

The professional view

In addition to best practice as described by EBN there is a regulatory or quality view of best practice as reflected by professional groups which deliver health care to children and families. This view of best practice is often reflected in professional standards, competencies and codes of practice (New Zealand Nurses Organisation 2012; Nursing and Midwifery Board New South Wales 2013; Registered Nurses' Association of Ontario

2008; Royal College of Nursing 2011), and may capture best practice from both the perspective of EBN and quality. However, the emphasis in this view of best practice is on describing the standards of best practice expected of nurses when working with children and families. While there may be some criticism that these standards, competencies and codes of practice are too generic and may not address the specialist nature of children's nursing, they are often the basis for registration and legal practice within countries. This is an aspect which nurses sometimes lose sight of in the busyness of practice, and it is often not until something goes wrong or a complaint is made by families that nurses become aware that practice has fallen below the standards expected.

The consumer view: children's and families' views

The final and perhaps most important view of best practice, which is often overlooked, is that described by the children and families who receive health care. The growth of health consumerism and the recognition that consumer perspectives are important to ensuring best practice has led to more emphasis being placed on capturing the child's and family's perspective (Boivin et al. 2010; Sajid and Baig 2007). In nursing, this perspective is frequently presented by parents who act as proxies for their children (Dickens et al. 2011; Latour et al. 2009). However, increasingly children are being given an opportunity to present their own views of what reflects best (or bad) practice (Coyne and Kirwan 2012; Jensen et al. 2012). Including the voice of children in measuring and determining best practice is becoming standard practice in many countries, particularly in the UK (Cavet and Sloper 2004; Coad et al. 2008), and there is a strong international call for children's right to participate. However, it is still not common international practice for child or family perspectives to be routinely incorporated into health service quality management systems, or to have children or families participating in clinical guidelines development. The family view of best practice is more frequently left to be represented by public media such as newspapers, television or parent advocacy groups. Parent advocacy groups such as Action for Children, Young People Aotearoa and Action for Sick Children have been particularly successful in influencing and changing practice.

While some views of best practice are more dominant within nursing, increasingly we are seeing the interplay between the various views of best practice. While this interplay can bring with it tensions and challenges, it perhaps provides the best opportunity to encapsulate a comprehensive view of best practice.

Case study 7.4: Beth

The perspective of the child and family

The perspectives of children, young people or families were not sought or represented in the development of the oral health guidelines or in the campaign at Beth's hospital. The nurses were not dismissive of a child and family perspective in the development of the guideline but they did not directly seek to determine child or family satisfaction with oral health care practices, either before or after the best practice guideline was implemented.

How do we know when practice is not 'the best'?

As we have seen in the previous section, there are various ways in which best practice is described but how do we know when practice is or is not at its best? Unfortunately, judgement of best practice is frequently made from a negative or deficit perspective. This is often represented by the reporting of a medical error or complaints made by children, families or the general public about service delivery. While there are acknowledged difficulties with the process of using medical error reporting and complaints systems (Allsop and Jones 2008; Evans et al. 2006), often the criteria used for judging the validity of the complaint is that of best practice. In many countries these systems may operate internally within the organisation, for example, via hospital complaints systems or externally via government and other professional bodies (http://www.hdc.org.nz/complaints/complaints-resolution-overview).

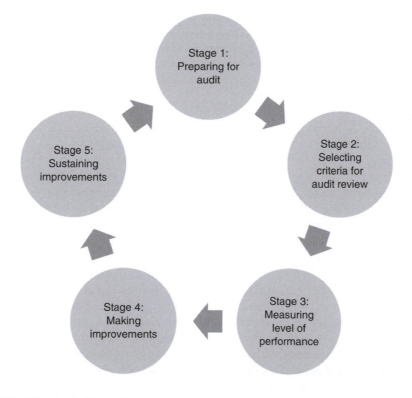

Figure 7.1   The Audit Cycle (Benjamin 2008)

A more proactive and positive approach to determining whether the practice within a health service reflects best practice is to undertake an evaluation or audit. This can be done using a research evaluation process or using the principles for quality audit highlighted in Figure 7.1 (Benjamin 2008).

Evaluation drawing on research principles is often undertaken when little is known about practice and you wish to generate information that can be applied or generalised to other health settings. These types of evaluations are frequently published in peer reviewed publications and reports. Quality audits, on the other hand, may be published (Crellin et al. 2010) but are often an internal process where practice is measured against proven standards of high quality care to bring practice into line with these standards so as to improve the quality of care and health (Brain et al. 2011).

Case study 7.5: Beth

Establishing the criteria for audit

In Beth's hospital little was known about current oral health practices in the hospital or how these compared with what was described in the literature and by the Ministry of Health as 'best practice'. This meant they began the project with a formal research evaluation (Dickinson et al. 2009). Once a best practice standard was established in the form of a clinical guideline they then audited the nurses' practice against the best practice guideline they had set (internal audit).

A less reliable way to determine the level of nursing care being delivered is to benchmark the care delivered in one hospital or health care service against that of others. One of the difficulties of using this approach is that interpretation of what is 'best practice' may be variable between services and may or may not reflect best practice as determined by the best evidence. However, this process is sometimes used when nurses are unable to locate higher levels of evidence to support practice or where they wish to improve performance (Kingston et al. 2010). In the absence of scientific evidence, regulatory and auditing bodies frequently determine best practice based on what is deemed acceptable by reputable and high-quality health services.

Best practice in caring for children and families can be viewed from a number of perspectives, these being: the scientific evidence; organisational government or professional standards regulations or codes of practice; and the perspectives of children and families. While there may be challenges to gaining a comprehensive view of best practice, all perspectives must be considered. Similarly, there are a number of ways in which best practice can be measured or evaluated and it is important that nurses consider which tools are appropriate, the benefits and limitations of each and how they, the families, colleagues, employers, providers and funders of health services may view and use such evaluations.

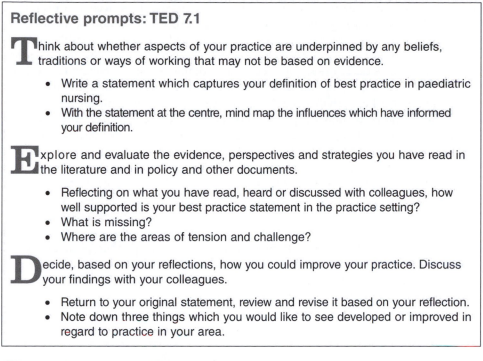

Reflective prompts: TED 7.1

Think about whether aspects of your practice are underpinned by any beliefs, traditions or ways of working that may not be based on evidence.

- Write a statement which captures your definition of best practice in paediatric nursing.
- With the statement at the centre, mind map the influences which have informed your definition.

Explore and evaluate the evidence, perspectives and strategies you have read in the literature and in policy and other documents.

- Reflecting on what you have read, heard or discussed with colleagues, how well supported is your best practice statement in the practice setting?
- What is missing?
- Where are the areas of tension and challenge?

Decide, based on your reflections, how you could improve your practice. Discuss your findings with your colleagues.

- Return to your original statement, review and revise it based on your reflection.
- Note down three things which you would like to see developed or improved in regard to practice in your area.

Changing practice

It is now widely recognised that developing evidence based guidelines and disseminating them into the practice area is not sufficient to bring about practice change. A carefully planned change process and implementation strategy must be in place to facilitate practice change. A range of models for changing practice have been put forward in nursing, some related directly to EBP (McCormack et al. 2002b; Stetler 2001; Titler 2007) while others draw on models from continuous quality improvement and management theory (Black and Brennan 2011; Brookes 2011; McLean 2011a, 2011b). All of the models note the importance of having a well-designed process for change alongside an awareness of the factors that might facilitate or act as barriers to changing practice.

A climate for change

In all of these models, change begins with an awareness of the need for practice to change. While most models describe this as the beginning point, McLean (2011b) put forward the idea that it is in fact an 'ending' in recognising that old ways of practising are no longer working. Change usually relates to a problem or failure of practice. Successful change is dependent on the organisation and those involved in the change recognising that practice needs to change. There is an extensive body of nursing literature which identifies the things which influence nurses' ability to consider implementing evidence based guidelines or changing practice, including: workload and exhaustion, attitude to and knowledge of research, lack of access to resources, time and lack of authority (Estabrooks 1999; Estabrooks et al. 2003). Most of the studies have operated from the premise that nurses will commit to an EBP approach and that it is the individual nurses' behaviour which will be responsible for the adoption of new practices. However, the focus on individual nurses' behaviour and the premise that one source of knowledge (scientific evidence) is sufficient to inform nursing practice is being challenged. Nurse authors are now recognising and suggesting that one source of knowledge may not be sufficient to ensure innovative and quality care. They note that there is an inextricable link between structural, organisational and social influences which impact on nurses' ability to change practice (Cummings et al. 2007; Estabrooks et al. 2005; Mantzoukas 2008; McCormack et al. 2002a; Titler 2007; Wall 2008). For nursing practice to develop, organisational values must be consistent with a culture of innovation, challenge and change. A climate for change is set when the health service recognises the facilitators and barriers to change, has strategies for strengthening or weakening their influence and values the contribution and leadership of all employees. There are a number of quality tools which can be used to assist nurses in understanding the facilitators of and barriers to change. Lewins Force Field Analysis (Baulcomb 2003) is one such tool which can easily be used in the practice setting (see Figure 7.2).

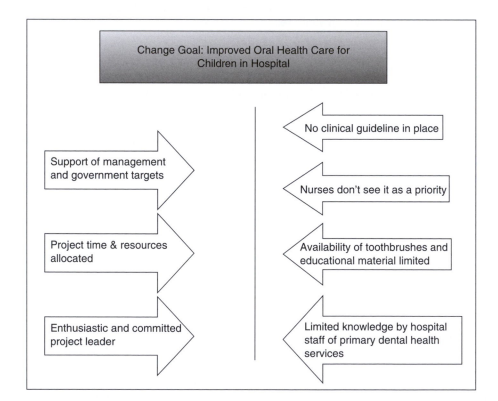

Figure 7.2 Force Field Analysis

Case study 7.6: Beth

The climate for change

Beth and the Nurse Director came to recognise the need to change practice. However, the impetus for changing or improving practice was largely driven by a government health target which had been imposed on her organisation. This 'top-down' approach may not have been the ideal basis for change. The responses from the PICU and Oncology Unit nurses suggest that there may not have been sufficient 'buy-in' for the need to change. While Beth and her team may have had the organisational support which is important to implement change, there did not appear to be sufficient recognition by the nurses and nurse managers in the clinical settings that practice needed to change. It appears that right from the outset while Beth, her manager, the organisation and the health ministry recognised the need for practice to change, there was insufficient discomfort amongst the nurses in the hospital to want to change.

A plan for change

The next important factor for successful practice change is to ensure that the implementation of the practice change is carefully planned. This includes the following factors: identification of the key stakeholders who can either facilitate or act as a barrier to change; selecting change leaders and champions who will facilitate the change; clearly communicating what is changing and why; selecting appropriate change strategies; and deciding what outcomes one expects from the practice change and how progress will be measured. McLean (2011b) also points to the need to assess the 'old' before creating the new to ensure that those things that are working well and are well supported by evidence are not abandoned but incorporated into the new way of practising.

Identifying and involving key stakeholders, effective leadership and having a team to champion the change are well recognised as key factors in successful change management, leadership being of particular importance. Two styles of leadership have been described within the change theory and practice development literature. The first, transactional leadership, is often dominant in hierarchical structures where there are rigid rules, standards and lines of command. Leaders using this style of leadership focus on tasks and getting compliance with standards and guidelines. While practice change can result from this type of leadership, it is the second form of leadership, transformational leadership, which has been linked in nursing to improving the quality of care delivered (Marchionni and Ritchie 2008a; McCormack et al. 2002a). Transformational leaders inspire staff to achieve a shared vision for quality health care, encourage challenges to the status quo and recognise the potential for all to participate and lead. They are open to using a wide range of strategies to implement change and are flexible and open to challenge. One of the difficulties is that often the structure of the organisation may not enable such leadership. Leaders operating in organisations which do not support transformational leaders must be willing to challenge, subvert or even work around environmental structures which may obstruct practice development.

Case study 7.7: Beth

Planning the change

Beth was chosen to lead the project because the Nurse Director recognised her potential as a transformational leader. While aspiring to innovation and shared leadership, the organisation to which Beth belonged held on to fairly tight hierarchal structures. Predetermined timeframes and targets and, to some degree, the processes and systems of the organisation, often challenged Beth's ability to operate in a transformational way. Despite this and with the support of the Nurse Director, Beth was able to set up a network of 'change champions' and these were valuable in the development of the best practice guideline and implementation of the practice change across services.

A clear communication strategy was established including hospital-wide education sessions. These education sessions were timed for maximum impact to occur at the same time as the National Children's Oral Health Care campaign was occurring within schools, primary health care services and in the media. A range of change strategies was used including resource kits, educational sessions, messages and prompts via email and the hospital intranet, as well as posters targeted at both nurses and families. It would have been difficult for nurses working in the hospital at the time to avoid knowing about the proposed change and expectations in regard to oral health care practices. Clear outcome measures were established based on the earlier baseline evaluation, clinical practice guideline and government targets. Children and families entering the service were expected to have an oral health care assessment using a predetermined tool, to receive regular oral care as described in the guideline, and be enrolled with the dental health service. Beth and her team had paid attention to the principles of good practice change so it was not unrealistic for them to expect results.

Responding to change

Unfortunately, developing and implementing a practice change does not in itself change practice, and this is due not only to the culture or climate within the organisation but also to how nurses, other health professionals and indeed the children and families themselves respond to the change. The Diffusion of Innovations model (Rogers 1995) has been widely used and adapted within health care settings to assist in understanding how innovation and practice change is adopted within health organisations. The key attributes of Diffusion of Innovation are:

- Relative advantage (is this practice better than what we have now?)
- Compatibility (does it fit within the practice setting?)
- Complexity (is it an easy practice to follow?)
- Triability (can we trial it before we decide to use it?)
- Observability (can we see and measure the results of the practice change?).

The characteristics of the participants and their responses to these questions therefore need to be considered, and while some individuals embrace change (early adopters), others struggle with and are often resistant to change (laggards) (Oldenburg and Glanz 2008). In some organisations change is happening so often and so frequently that nurses become exhausted by the change and take a stance described by McLean (2011a) as 'change blindness', this occurs when they decide to ignore the change and carry on as usual hoping it will never happen. Practice change is a challenging and anxious time for those involved. Anxiety and stress are inherent within practice development, particularly during the time of transition when the new practice has not been fully embedded within practice. Nurses need to be supported during times of change and their discomfort with change needs to be acknowledged. It is important that communication systems are strong. The change team needs to continue to promote the change in relation to how it will benefit children and families and to be open and adaptable to considering the suggestions and concerns of the nurses.

The term 'tipping point' has often been used as a popular way of describing the point at which there is sufficient 'buy-in' by the team to the practice change so that it will no longer be a 'new' practice but become embedded 'as practice'. However, this is, as Oldenburg and Glanz (2008) note, dependent on the factors already mentioned, including: having influential early adopters or 'champions'; presenting a change which has qualities and attributes which are compelling; and having environmental factors in place which support the change. An understanding of these concepts and responses not only assists nurses in planning change and supporting the team through the change but also provides a framework to reflect on why, despite the best plans, practice change does not always happen.

Case study 7.8: Beth

Diffusion of Innovation

Beth had already noted that the nurses in her organisation had difficulty identifying the need to change so it became difficult to argue relative advantage. While at a higher level no one could argue against the need to improve the oral health of the children in the country, the nurses were not convinced that their individual practice could influence this. The oral health care project and campaign was primarily a nursing initiative, the influence of other members of the interdisciplinary team and, in fact, the children and families themselves received minimal attention. While the nursing staff might embrace the notion of health promotion and delivery of effective oral care to children within both acute and primary health care settings, if other members of the team did not see it as a priority, particularly highly influential stakeholders such as paediatricians and parents, then the practice change would be difficult to implement. The notion of compatibility of preventative health promotion strategy within an acute paediatric hospital was not addressed. A dominant driver for this practice change was health service targets rather than a discomfort of the nurses with practice. The timeframes placed around the project provided little opportunity to trial the change prior to full implementation; although there was the ability to change and adapt the practice change as it was implemented this did not entirely meet the needs of trialability as

(Continued)

(Continued)

described in the Diffusion of Innovation model. Observability was addressed by Beth and her team by audits and surveys throughout the change process. However, the expected outcomes and the timeframe given to achieve these may have been set too high given the nature of the practice change and the complexity of the health service in which it was being introduced. For Beth and her team the expectation that the practice change would be fully implemented within six months was unrealistic, and while practice had not changed measurably there were indicators that practice was changing.

For practice change to be successful it must be widely visible across the organisation via posters, promotion packs and educational activities. Team review, audits and benchmarking are also important so that the nurses and other team members receive regular feedback and can measure the change; this is part of the essential feedback loop (McCormack et al. 2002b). As Marchionni and Ritchie (2008b) suggest, nurses often overestimate the magnitude of practice change they expect to see.

In this section we have seen that the identification of best practice is but the first step in ensuring that children and families receive quality care. While in some instances the

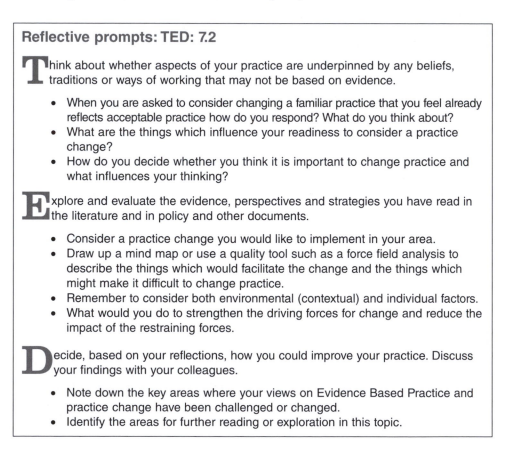

Reflective prompts: TED: 7.2

Think about whether aspects of your practice are underpinned by any beliefs, traditions or ways of working that may not be based on evidence.

- When you are asked to consider changing a familiar practice that you feel already reflects acceptable practice how do you respond? What do you think about?
- What are the things which influence your readiness to consider a practice change?
- How do you decide whether you think it is important to change practice and what influences your thinking?

Explore and evaluate the evidence, perspectives and strategies you have read in the literature and in policy and other documents.

- Consider a practice change you would like to implement in your area.
- Draw up a mind map or use a quality tool such as a force field analysis to describe the things which would facilitate the change and the things which might make it difficult to change practice.
- Remember to consider both environmental (contextual) and individual factors.
- What would you do to strengthen the driving forces for change and reduce the impact of the restraining forces.

Decide, based on your reflections, how you could improve your practice. Discuss your findings with your colleagues.

- Note down the key areas where your views on Evidence Based Practice and practice change have been challenged or changed.
- Identify the areas for further reading or exploration in this topic.

identification of best practice may validate current practice, in most instances nurses will be required to change their practice and this can be an anxious and stressful time. Practice development therefore requires careful planning and recognition of how the process of change and responses to the change may influence the effectiveness of implementing best practice. A number of implementation models from EBP and quality improvement and management theory provide useful frameworks to guide nurses leading and participating in practice development.

Creating and maintaining a culture of best practice

Nurses are increasingly expected to lead and maintain nursing practices which meet professional standards (as determined by the profession), reflect government policy and health targets, are evidence based (research driven), are effective and efficient in their delivery and use of health resources, and are measurable in relation to health outcomes for children and families. This is within the context of rapid advancement in technologies and treatments, complex and diverse health delivery systems, changes in skill mix including non-regulated workers, variability in relation to access to and availability of health resources and professional development opportunities, consumerism, and the changing nature of illness and health across and within countries. The question may be asked as to whether best practice can be maintained at all times and whether EBP and practice development make a difference to children and families? This section will consider the actual and potential outcomes of 'best practice' and what is required if a culture of best practice is to be created and maintained.

There is some evidence that developing best practice guidelines and implementing them in practice can change practice but more limited evidence to support an improvement in patient outcomes. For example, Black and Brennan (2011) demonstrated that one year after implementation of a bronchiolitis protocol there was an increase in nurses' use of the suction protocol, a decrease in use of Beta2-agonisists, a decrease in mean length of stay and a decrease in medical costs. Randhawa et al. (2010) demonstrated that three years after implementation of a Pediatric Early Warning Score (PEWS) there was a reduction in cardiopulmonary arrests and an improvement in the early detection skills of bedside nurses. Thomas et al. (2010) reported improved efficiency of administration of comfort measures to children in a Paediatric Intensive Care Unit (PICU) in Canada three months after the introduction of a Sedation and Analgesic Guideline.

The most frequently used criteria for measuring success are changes in nurses' or health professionals' behaviours, use of health services or the financial advantage to the health service. The impact and outcomes for children and families are often not measured or reported. So while we might equate reduction in length of stay, use of validated assessment tools, more effective use of treatments or drugs and referral to appropriate health services and professionals as having beneficial outcomes for children and families, longitudinal robust evidence in this area remains limited.

Creating and maintaining an environment of best practice in children's nursing requires close linkages between clinicians and researchers and nurses, who are strong research consumers. One of the difficulties that clinicians face is that often when they attempt to seek out research which supports and guides practice they are unable to locate the evidence they need. This may relate to two factors. Firstly, the number of research units and researchers engaged in clinical nursing research remains small and under-resourced, and secondly, the research that nurses engage in is not producing the answers to the clinical questions clinicians seek. If children and families are to receive the best care there needs to be strong linkages between nurse researchers and clinicians so that not only does research inform practice but practice informs the research undertaken. While a number of successful models of achieving this have been put forward, including clinical research nurses (Currey et al. 2011), clinical academic partnerships (Sigsworth 2009), practice development units (Appleton et al. 2010) and Clinical Academic Training Pathways (NHS National Institute of Health Research 2013), significant challenges remain in relation to competing demands and resourcing and sustaining strong research and clinical links (Darbyshire, 2010).

Another important factor in creating and maintaining a culture of best practice is to have supportive policies (local and national) and organisations which demand, encourage and resource innovation and the translation of research in practice. As previously discussed in this chapter, the influence of contextual and environmental factors on developing and ensuring best practice has been well studied. We also now have evidence from the studies related to Magnet® hospitals that both patient and nursing outcomes can be improved when environments conducive to innovation are created. Magnet® hospitals are hospitals which are recognised by the American Nurses Credentialing Center (ANCC) as delivering excellent patient outcomes, having high levels of nurse job satisfaction, a low nursing staff turnover rate and high level of nursing involvement in the decision-making regarding the delivery of care. While the original Magnet® work is now over 20 years old, subsequent studies continue to note that better work environments, more highly educated nurses, high levels of autonomy and positive nurse–physician relationships result in significantly better nurse outcomes (Barton et al. 2012; Kelly et al. 2011; Laschinger et al. 2003). However, the policy and organisational support has to extend throughout all levels of the health service.

Another factor key to the successful creation of a culture of best practice is to have robust linkages between EBP and organisational systems, particularly quality management systems (Rycroft-Malone et al., 2004, Titler, 2007, Titler et al., 2001). This encourages not only attention to outcomes, audit and review but also provides the vehicle to implement and establish practice change.

As discussed earlier in the chapter, strong nursing leadership is the key to creating and maintaining a culture of innovation and best practice. Nursing requires leaders who can inspire, challenge and support nurses in engaging in practice development. Nurse leaders need to be willing to advocate strongly within their organisations for resources and structures which support innovation and practice development. The notion of transformational leadership has been put forward, but to develop such leadership requires not only organisations which support this form of leadership, but also nurses who are willing to engage and be transformed. No matter how strong the leadership is, unless nurses regularly review and develop their own practice we cannot hope to improve health service delivery and outcomes for children and families. Nurses can develop their practice through being open to review by others, willing to engage with the professional debate and research in their area of practice and willing to consider innovative ways of doing things.

A culture of best practice will only be developed and maintained if nurses are willing to take responsibility for the care that is delivered to children in their unit or services. Nurses should never condone or ignore care which falls below acceptable standards. Unfortunately, sometimes nurses are unwilling to challenge the practice of their colleagues; the reasons for this may vary, from fear of reprisals, fear of the consequences to themselves and the nurse involved and the impact on relationships within the team and the manager's response. Nurses often operate in very hierarchical structures, which may mean that they perceive it is not their role to critique the practice of colleagues. Power differences between junior and senior staff can make it difficult for junior nurses to challenge the practice of a more senior or more experienced colleague (Dickinson et al. 2010). As previously discussed, the influence of the environment is significant. In environments which are transformative and empowering, supportive peer review and critique are enabled. In more hierarchical and 'blaming' environments, practice development becomes more challenging. Often, however, nurses' failure to act or intervene relates to their lack of skill and confidence in providing supportive critical peer critique. For a culture of best practice to exist, nurses must be educated and supported in developing the communication skills and techniques needed to enable collegial challenge and critique of practice.

A final area which still requires considerable attention is ensuring that we engage children and families in real and effective ways of determining best practice and how this can most effectively be delivered. We have seen the development internationally of charters which call for participation of children and families in clinical decision making and determining how services should be developed and delivered (Children's Hospitals Australasia and the Paediatric Society of New Zealand 2010; Royal College of Paediatrics and Child Health 2013) and have some examples of how this can be effectively done (Macdonald et al. 2007; Maynard et al. 2005). However, the voice of the professional or experts remains dominant in determining what is best practice. If we wish to aspire to providing the very best care to children and families we must not only provide the structures for them to regularly engage but also the robust tools and strategies which enable them to work collaboratively in determining a culture of best practice.

What is becoming clearer from the evaluations of practice developments and implementation of evidence based guidelines is that creating and maintaining a culture of innovation and change in practice are reliant on factors including strong linkages between researchers and clinicians, supportive government and organisational policies, and procedures which encourage and demand innovation and practice development. Also required are strong and robust quality management systems, transformational leadership, nurses who are effective users of research and who are willing to challenge, be challenged and change, and a willingness to engage with the consumers of care – children and families.

Creating and maintaining a 'change' culture and culture of best practice will continue to be challenging within an increasingly global, dynamic and complex health and nursing environment. The demand for change is constant and, with the development of

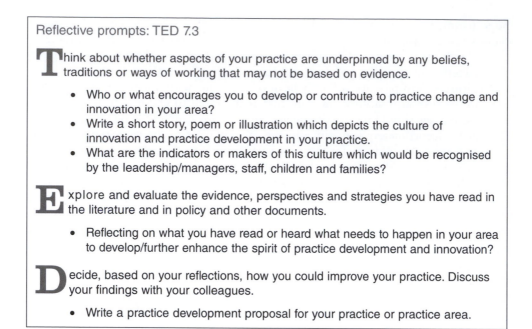

Reflective prompts: TED 7.3

Think about whether aspects of your practice are underpinned by any beliefs, traditions or ways of working that may not be based on evidence.

- Who or what encourages you to develop or contribute to practice change and innovation in your area?
- Write a short story, poem or illustration which depicts the culture of innovation and practice development in your practice.
- What are the indicators or makers of this culture which would be recognised by the leadership/managers, staff, children and families?

Explore and evaluate the evidence, perspectives and strategies you have read in the literature and in policy and other documents.

- Reflecting on what you have read or heard what needs to happen in your area to develop/further enhance the spirit of practice development and innovation?

Decide, based on your reflections, how you could improve your practice. Discuss your findings with your colleagues.

- Write a practice development proposal for your practice or practice area.

information technologies, will be increasingly rapid. Often one innovation or practice development is not fully embedded before there is a demand for another. This is demanding of nursing time, energy and resources, and therefore one can understand nurses' decisions to ignore or refuse to engage in practice development. There is comfort and security in old and familiar practices and, in an increasingly complex and demanding work environment, such familiarity is attractive. However, a culture of innovation and change can also energise and motivate nurses to find new and exciting ways of improving the health and well-being of children and families. Developing and improving practice will never be easy, but it must and should remain central to nursing practice.

Conclusion

Identifying and developing best practice is central to the care of children and young people. While the notion of 'best practice' within nursing is often viewed from the dominant research based perspective, this chapter has challenged the reader to consider a wider perspective which incorporates perspectives of quality and risk, professional standards and, most importantly, that of children and their families. In this chapter it has been argued that defining best practice is just a foundation for the more challenging task of changing and transforming practice. Challenges and influences on the change process have been reviewed alongside the factors which might influence nurses' engagement in developing practice. In an increasingly global and complex health environment where the demand for change is constant, innovation and development will be central to ensuring that the care delivered to children and families is not only safe but of the highest quality.

References

Allsop, J. and Jones, K. (2008) 'Withering the citizen, managing the consumer: complaints in healthcare settings', *Social Policy and Society*, 7: 233–243.

Appleton, L., Smith, K. and Wyatt, D. (2010) 'Nursing involvement in a practice development and research unit', *Cancer Nursing Practice*, 9: 18–22.

Barton, S.J., Forster, E.K., Stuart, M.E., Patton, A.M., Rim, J.-S. and Torowicz, D.L. (2012) 'New knowledge, innovations, and improvement in a Magnet® Children's Hospital Cardiac Center', *Journal of Pediatric Nursing*, 27: 271–274.

Baulcomb, J.S. (2003) 'Management of change through force field analysis', *Journal of Nursing Management*, 11: 275–280.

Benjamin, A. (2008) 'Audit: how to do it in practice', *British Medical Journal*, 336: 1241–1245.

Black, A. and Brennan, R. A. (2011) 'Breathing easy: implementing a bronchiolitis protocol', *Pediatric Nursing*, 37: 129–135.

Boivin, A., Currie, K., Fervers, B., Gracia, J., James, M., Marshall, C., Sakala, C., Sanger, S., Strid, J., Thomas, V., Van Der Weijden, T., Grol, R. and Burgers, J. (2010) 'Patient and public involvement in clinical guidelines: international experiences and future perspectives', *Quality and Safety in Health Care*, 19: 1–4.

Brain, J., Schofield, J., Gerrish, K., Mawson, S., Mabbott, I., Patel, D. and Gerrish, P. (2011) *A Guide to Clinical Audit, Research and Service Review – An Educational Toolkit Designed to Help Staff Differentiate Between Clinical Audit, Research and Service Review Activities.* Sheffield: HQIP.

Brookes, J. (2011) 'Engaging staff in the change process', *Nursing Management*, 18: 16–19.

Cavet, J. and Sloper, P. (2004) 'The participation of children and young people in decisions about UK service development', *Child: Care, Health & Development*, 30: 613–621.

Children's Hospitals Australasia and the Paediatric Society of New Zealand (2010) *Charter on the Rights of Tamariki Children & Rangatahi Young People in Healthcare Services in Aotearoa New Zealand.* Wellington: Children's Hospitals Australasia.

Coad, J., Flay, J., Aspinall, M., Bilverstone, B., Coxhead, E. and Hones, B. (2008) 'Evaluating the impact of involving young people in developing children's services in an acute hospital trust', *Journal of Clinical Nursing*, 17: 3115–3122.

Coyne, I. and Kirwan, L. (2012) 'Ascertaining children's wishes and feelings about hospital life', *Journal of Child Health Care*, 16: 293–304.

Crellin, D., Catling, S., Carter, A., Alexander, S., Ryan, S. and Pang, P.Y. (2010) 'Audit of paediatric forearm plasters: adherence to discharge education and referral recommendations', *Australasian Emergency Nursing Journal*, 13: 135.

Cummings, G., Estabrooks, C., Midodzi, W., Wallin, L. and Hayduk, L. (2007) 'Influence of organizational characteristics and context on research utilization', *Nursing Research*, 56: S24–39.

Currey, J., Considine, J. and Khaw, D. (2011) 'Clinical nurse research consultant: a clinical and academic role to advance practice and the discipline of nursing', *Journal of Advanced Nursing*, 67: 2275–2283.

Darbyshire, P. (2010) 'Joint or clinical chairs in nursing: from cup of plenty to poisoned chalice?', *Journal of Advanced Nursing*, 66: 2592–2599.

Dickens, K., Matthews, L.R. and Thompson, J. (2011) 'Parent and service providers' perceptions regarding the delivery of family-centred paediatric rehabilitation services in a children's hospital', *Child: Care, Health & Development*, 37: 64–73.

Dickinson, A., Mccall, E., Twomey, B. and James, N. (2010) 'Pediatric nurses' understanding of the process and procedure of double-checking medications', *Journal of Clinical Nursing*, 19: 728–735.

Dickinson, A., Peacock, K., Fair, N., Thomas, M., Nicol, R., Mikkelsen, J., Haselmore, J., Chapman, L., Garrett, N. and Johnstone, L. (2009) 'The implementation and evaluation of an oral healthcare best practice guideline in a paediatric hospital', *International Journal of Evidence-Based Healthcare*, 7: 34–42.

Estabrooks, C.A. (1999) 'Modeling the individual determinants of research utilization', *Western Journal of Nursing Research*, 21: 758–772.

Estabrooks, C.A., Floyd, J.A., Scott-Findlay, S., O'Leary, K.A. and Gushta, M. (2003) 'Individual determinants of research utilization: a systematic review', *Journal of Advanced Nursing*, 43: 506–520.

Estabrooks, C.A., Rutakumwa, W., O'Leary, K.A., Profetto-McGrath, J., Milner, M., Levers, M.J. and Scott-Findlay, S. (2005) 'Sources of practice knowledge among nurses', *Qualitative Health Research*, 15: 460–476.

Evans, S.M., Berry, J.G., Smith, B.J., Esterman, A., Selim, P., O'Shaughnessy, J. and Dewit, M. (2006) 'Attitudes and barriers to incident reporting: a collaborative hospital study', *Quality and Safety in Health Care*, 15: 39–43.

Jensen, C.S., Jackson, K., Kolbæk, R. and Glasdam, S. (2012) 'Children's experiences of acute hospitalisation to a paediatric emergency and assessment unit – a qualitative study', *Journal of Child Health Care*, 16: 263–273.

Kelly, L.A., McHugh, M.D. and Aiken, L.H. (2011) 'Nurse outcomes in Magnet® and non-magnet hospitals', *Journal of Nursing Administration*, 41: 428–433.

Kingston, F., Bryant, T. and Speer, K. (2010) 'Paediatric falls benchmarking collaborative', *Journal of Nursing Management*, 40: 287–292.

Laschinger, H.K., Almost, J. and Tuer-Hodes, D. (2003) 'Workplace empowerment and Magnet® hospital characteristics', *Journal of Nursing Administration*, 33: 410–422.

Latour, J.M., Goudoever, J.B., Duivenvoorden, H.J., van Dam, N.A., Dullaart, E., Albers, M.J.I.J., Verlaat, C.W.M., Vught, E.M., Heerde, M. and Hazelzet, J.A. (2009) 'Perceptions of parents on satisfaction with care in the pediatric intensive care unit: the EMPATHIC study', *Intensive Care Medicine*, 35: 1082–1089.

Macdonald, E.L., Geraghty, E., McCann, K., Mohay, H. and O'Brien, T. (2007) 'Towards a developmental framework of consumer and carer participation in child and adolescent mental health services', *Australasian Psychiatry*, 15: 504–508.

Mantzoukas, S. (2008) 'A review of evidence-based practice, nursing research and reflection: levelling the hierarchy', *Journal of Clinical Nursing*, 17: 214–223.

Marchionni, C. and Ritchie, J. (2008a) 'Organizational factors that support the implementation of a nursing best practice guideline', *Journal of Nursing Management*, 16: 266–274.

Marchionni, C. and Ritchie, J. (2008b) 'Organizational factors that support the implementation of a nursing Best Practice Guideline', *Journal of Nursing Management*, 16: 266–274.

Maynard, L., Rennie, T., Shirtliffe, J. and Vickers, D. (2005) 'Seeking and using families' views to shape children's hospice services', *International Journal of Palliative Nursing*, 11: 624–630.

McCormack, B., Kitson, A., Harvey, G., Rycroft-Malone, J., Titchen, A. and Seers, K. (2002a) 'Getting evidence into practice: the meaning of "context"', *Journal of Advanced Nursing*, 38: 94–104.

McCormack, B., Kitson, A., Harvey, G., Rycroft-Malone, J., Titchen, A. and Seers, K. (2002b) 'Getting evidence into practice: the meaning of "context"', *Journal of Advanced Nursing*, 38: 94–104.

McLean, C. (2011a) 'Change and transition: navigating the journey, *British Journal of School Nursing*, 6: 141–145.

McLean, C. (2011b) 'Change and transition: what is the difference?', *British Journal of School Nursing*, 6: 78–81.

Ministry of Health (2004) *Keep Me Smiling 'Lift the Lip': Early Identification of Tooth Decay in Infants and Children*. Wellington: Ministry of Health.

New Zealand Nurses Organisation (2012) *Guidelines for Nurses on the Administration of Medicines*. Wellington: New Zealand Nurses Organisation.

NHS National Institute of Health Research (2013) *Clinical Academic Training Programme for Nurses, Midwives and Allied Health Professionals*. National Institute of Health Research. Available at: http://www.nihrtcc.nhs.uk/cat/ (accessed 21 April 2013).

Nursing and Midwifery Board New South Wales (2013) *Professional Standards*. Nursing and Midwifery Board New South Wales. Available at: http://nursesstaging.elcom.com.au/professional-standards/default.aspx (accessed 18 April 2013).

Oldenburg, B. and Glanz, K. (2008) 'Diffusion of innovations', in K. Glanz, B.K. Rimer and K. Viswanath (eds) *Health Behavior and Health Education*, 4th edn. San Francisco: Jossey-Bass.

Pearson, A., Wiechula, R., Court, A. and Lockwood, C. (2005) 'The JBI model of evidence-based healthcare', *International Journal of Evidence-Based Healthcare*, 3: 207–215.

Randhawa, S., Roberts-Truner, R., Woronick, K. and Duval, J. (2010) 'Implementing and sustaining evidence-based practice to reduce pediatric cardiopulmonary arrest', *Western Journal of Nursing Research*, 33 443–456.

Registered Nurses' Association of Ontario (2008) 'Oral health: nursing assessment and interventions', *Nursing Best Practice Guidelines Program*. Toronto: Registered Nurses' Association of Ontario.

Rogers, D.M. (1995) *Diffusion of Innovation*. New York: Free Press.

Royal College of Nursing (2011) *Health Care Nursing Standards for Caring for Neonates, Children and Young People*. London: Royal College of Nursing.

Royal College of Paediatrics and Child Health (2013) *Standards of Care*. Royal College of Paediatrics and Child Health. Available at: www.rcpch.ac.uk/child-health/standards-care/standards-care (Accessed 21 April 2013).

Rycroft-Malone, J., Harvey, G., Seers, K., Kitson, A., McCormack, B. and Titchen, A. (2004) 'An exploration of the factors that influence the implementation of evidence into practice', *Journal of Clinical Nursing*, 13: 913–924.

Sajid, M.S. and Baig, M.K. (2007) 'Quality of health care: an absolute necessity for public satisfaction', *International Journal of Health Care Quality Assurance*, 20: 545–548.

Scott, K. and McSherry, R. (2009) 'Evidence-based nursing: clarifying the concepts for nurses in practice', *Journal of Clinical Nursing*, 18: 1085–1095.

Sigsworth, J. (2009) 'Bridging the gap between research and practice', *Nursing Management – UK*, 16: 20–22.

Stetler, C. (2001) 'Updating the Stetler Model of research utilization to facilitate evidence-based practice', *Nursing Outlook*, 49: 272–279.

Thomas, M., Dhanani, S., Irwin, D., Writer, H. and Doherty, D. (2010) 'Development, dissemination and implementation of a sedation and analgesic guideline in a pediatric intensive care unit ... it takes creativity and collaboration', *Dynamics: The Official Journal of the Canadian Association of Nurses*, 21: 16–25.

Titler, M. (2007) 'Translating research into practice', *American Journal of Nursing*, 107: 26–33.

Titler, M., Kleiber, C., Steelman, V., Rakel, B., Budreau, G., Everett, L., Buckwalter, K., Tripp-Reimer, T. and Goode, C. (2001) 'The Iowa Model of evidence-based practice to promote quality care', *Critical Care Nursing Clinics of North America*, 13: 497–509.

Wall, S. (2008) 'A critique of evidence-based practice in nursing: challenging the assumptions', *Social Theory & Health*, 6: 37–53.

Closing Thoughts: Celebrating Success and Aspiring for Better

There is much to celebrate within children's health care and the role that nurses have in caring for children, young people and their families. Nurses and other health professionals strive to improve services, outcomes and children's and their families' experiences; it is a shame that these achievements rarely make headlines. Unfortunately, the successes are often overshadowed by negative aspects of provision such as inequalities in access to services, incidents of poor care and failing systems. Adopting a critical stance, thinking clearly, robustly and passionately about our practice means we need to make time to stop and take a critical look at where we have come from and where we are in relation to the care that we provide to children. We need to ensure that as we step forward, the steps we take are ones which will take us in the right direction.

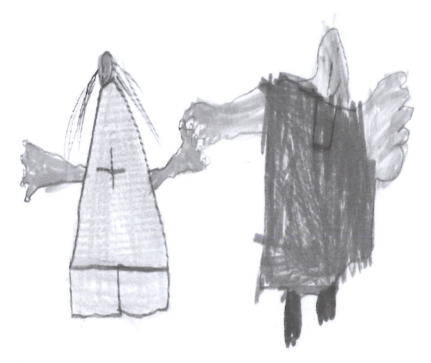

Figure CT.1 Children's nurse and child

The landscape of care has changed from the time when children were institutionalised and isolated within stark hospital environments. Some children, particularly those with disabilities in developing countries, continue to experience institutionalised care (United Nations Children's Fund 2013). However, in developed countries children and young people are being increasingly cared for within their own homes and in accessible short-stay services based on the recognition that being 'at home' and 'with my family' are usually the best place for children to be. Children in developing countries also experience illness and care within the home environment, but this is often as a result of a lack of accessible services and treatments, rather than as a choice. Advances in health care are evident through children and young people having access to an increased number of treatments and technologies to sustain and improve their lives; diseases which previously resulted in children dying are now often treatable. However, there are massive inequities in access to treatment and many children across the globe die as a result of preventable diseases. The increasing success in treating previously life threatening conditions means that some children and young people have to adapt to life with multiple conditions, ongoing treatment and bodies that function and appear 'different' to those of their peers. Parents, professionals, services and communities can facilitate and nurture these children and their families as they grow and support them in achieving their boundless potential.

The UN Convention on the Rights of the Child (1989) was ratified by most countries and the rights continue to inform the services for children and young people. These rights are summarised as:

- The right to a childhood
- The right to be educated
- The right to be healthy
- The right to be treated fairly
- The right to be heard

Even though published over 20 years ago, these rights are still not afforded to all children; some children continue to suffer from poverty, homelessness, abuse, neglect and preventable diseases (UNICEF 2013). Children and young people continue to experience poor health, often from preventable illnesses resulting from unhealthy life choices such as obesity and smoking in developed countries (Department of Health 2013) and preventable and treatable illnesses such as measles, pneumonia and diarrhoea in developing countries (Lozano et al. 2013; Bhutta et al. 2013; Fischer et al. 2013). Children and young people from disadvantaged backgrounds and those with disabilities face the poorest health outcomes (D'Souza et al. 2012; Craig et al. 2012; Department of Health 2013). These inequities persist despite being recognised for many years and being the focus of the first human rights treaty of the 21st century (United Nations 2006). Children and young people continue to experience challenges in how they are afforded their right to be physically, emotionally and psychosocially healthy.

One of the key rights from the UNCRC (1989) relates to a child's right to be heard. A key focus of this book has been on the importance of placing children at the centre of their care and recognising their competence to report and be involved in decisions about their lives and treatment. This book has critically discussed many key aspects which influence the care of children, young people and their families. Although children's and young people's engagement with parents, society, health professionals and services has changed from being 'seen and not heard' to increasingly recognised as competent reporters of their own lives, there is still much to do before they are afforded a voice which is consistently listened to and respected within many services. We propose that it is not enough for children to be heard, they must be listened to and their opinions, concerns, preferences and experiences respected and acted upon.

The opportunities for children and young people to achieve their aspirations are greater than at any other point in history. This also reflects the experiences of children and young people with long-term conditions and disabilities. In order for children to grow through adolescence into adulthood and fulfil their potential and aspirations they must be nurtured by an integrated education, health and social system working with them and their families at the centre. Within these systems, children and young people have a right to be cared for by people who are appropriately educated (World Health Organization 2003). Services must take a life-course approach, coherently addressing children's and young people's issues, now and in the future based on their history and experiences instead of tackling individual aspects of the child's body and condition. Nurses are in a privileged position to be able to promote and support children and young people in making decisions and choices about their lives and health care, which will equip them for the decisions and choices that will be expected of them as they become young adults.

Although working with children and young people can be complex, difficult, and challenging, we believe and know that it is also eminently rewarding, exciting and illuminating. We support the key recommendation of the Children and Young People's Health Outcomes Forum in the UK (Department of Health 2013) which states that children, young people and their families should be at the heart of what happens. We hope this book has informed and inspired you to re-examine those often taken for granted aspects of practice which if questioned and changed have the potential to improve the outcomes and experiences of children, young people and their families.

We present an aspirational set of goals based on our shared and critical consideration of what should underpin the health care of all children and young people. We do not present these in any particular order of priority, they are all important and all deserve our attention.

- All children and young people should be cared for within the context of their family.
- All children and young people should be cared for in a way which values and respects the values and culture of their family and community.
- All children and young people should be cared for in a way that centres attention on their particular needs, strengths and circumstances.
- All children and young people should be listened to and heard.
- All children and young people should be supported to express their concerns, opinions and perspectives in a way to suit their preferences and abilities.
- No child or young person should suffer from treatable pain or other symptoms of illness.

- No child or young person should be without comfort.
- No child or young person should suffer from a preventable illness.
- Every child and young person's best interests should be respected, protected and advocated for.
- All children and young people should receive care in a space and place that best suits their needs and those of their family.
- All children and young people should be cared for by informed, passionate and appropriately trained professionals.
- No child or young person should be uncertain or unknowing, unless expressly chosen, of their condition, illness or planned treatment.
- All children and young people should receive high quality and safe care based on evidence and best practice.
- All children and young people should have access to services to promote and support their health.

References

Bhutta, Z.A., Das, J.K., Walker, N., Rizvi, A., Campbell, H., Rudan, I. and Black, R.E. (2013) 'Interventions to address deaths from childhood pneumonia and diarrhoea equitably: What works and at what cost?', *The Lancet*, 381(9875): 1417–29.

Craig, E., Mcdonald, G., Adams, J., Reddington, A., Oben, G., Simpson, J. and Wicken, A. (2012) *Te Ohonga Ake:The Health of Māori Children and Young People with Chronic Conditions and Disabilities in New Zealand*. Wellington: New Zealand Child and Youth Epidemiology Service for Ministry of Health.

Department of Health (2013) *Improving Children and Young People's Health Outcomes: A System Wide Response*. London: Department of Health.

D'Souza, A.J., Turner, N., Simmers, D., Craig, E. and Dowell, T. (2012) 'Every child to thrive, belong and achieve? Time to reflect and act in New Zealand', *New Zealand Medical Journal*, 125(1352).

Fischer Walker, C.L., Munos, M.K. and Black, R.E. (2013) 'Quantifying the indirect effects of key child survival interventions for pneumonia, diarrhoea, and measles', *Epidemiology and Infection*, 141(1): 115–31.

Lozano, R., Naghavi, M., Foreman, K., et al. (2013) 'Global and regional mortality from 235 causes of death for 20 age groups in 1990 and 2010: a systematic analysis for the Global Burden of Disease Study 2010', *The Lancet*, 380(9859): 2095–128.

United Nations (1989) *Convention on the Rights of the Child*. New York: United Nations General Assembly.

United Nations (2006) *Convention on the Rights of Persons with Disabilities*. Geneva: United Nations.

United Nations Children's Fund (2013) *State of the World's Children. Children with Disabilities*. New York: UNICEF

World Health Organization (2003) *WHO Europe Children's Nursing Curriculum. WHO European Strategy for Continuing Education for Nurses and Midwives*. Geneva: World Health Organization.

Index

advocacy groups 154
advocacy 4, 41, 117, 151, 154
advocacy role 41, 78, 91
age 123
  competency 80–1
  of majority 79
Alderson, P. 78, 79, 80–1, 88, 90
Allen, D. 28–9
American Nurses Credentialing Center
  (ANCC) 164
Andrews, G. J. 98
anxiety
  decision making 77–8
  hospital treatments 133
  procedures 64–5
  script theory 66
  timing of information 67
arts-based methods 46
assent 11, 31, 50, 75, 80, 88–90, 91, 93, 94
Association for the Wellbeing of Children in
  Healthcare (AWCH) 14
asthma 43, 47, 59, 61, 63, 86, 122, 123,
  125–6, 128
  internet information 63
  research 43, 47
  toolkit 59
  written information 61
Attention Deficit Hyperactivity Disorder
  (ADHD) 46–7
audio recordings 60–1
audit 164
  cycle 155–6
Australian National Standards for Children and
  Adolescents in Health Care 15
Australian Paediatric Association 19
autonomy 28, 75, 83, 84, 164

Bacigalupe, G. 103, 104
Baines, P. 84
Baulcomb, J. S. 158
behaviourism 36
Bellamy, C. 36–7
benchmarks 156
Bender, A. 108, 109
Berman, H. 124

best interests 13, 15, 25, 40, 41, 78, 84, 174
'best interests of the child' 41, 84
best practice 4, 5, 6, 10, 28, 149,
  150–66
Black, A. 163
Black, B. 4
Borglin, G. 4
boundaries, spaces 113–15
Bray, L. 55, 56, 57, 61, 67, 68, 77–8, 82, 85,
  86–90
Brennan, R. A. 163
Bristol Inquiry Report 14, 29, 54–5
bronchiolitis 122, 163
Buckley, A. 133

Callery, P. 25, 43, 58, 59, 65, 85, 129
cancer 61, 125, 126–7, 133–5, 136, 137
  decision making 77
  fatigue 137
carers 6, 24, 25, 28, 35, 40, 42, 97, 104, 107,
  108, 109, 129
Carter, B. 3, 19, 22, 25, 26, 45, 46, 47, 58, 106,
  107, 111, 122, 128, 137, 138, 139
Castle, K. 138
cerebral palsy 97–8, 105–6
change blindness 161
change management 159–63
Chan, Z. C. Y. 5
Charter on the Rights of Children and Young
  People in Health Care Services in Australia 81
The Charter on the Rights of Tamariki Children
  and Rangatahi Young People in Healthcare
  Services in Aotearoa New Zealand 26
chemotherapy 134–5
Chester, J. 14
child-centred 3, 6, 9, 14, 14, 25, 26, 27, 28, 35,
  42, 43, 45
child-centred care (CCC) 9–10,
  24–8, 35
child-centred research 35, 42, 43, 45, 46
child participation 9, 26, 44
childhood 36, 37, 38
children's wards 11–13
Children and Young People's Health Outcomes
  Forum 173

children with disabilities
  decision making 91
  treatment participation 40
Chimney Sweeps Act 1840 36
choice(s) 6, 17, 22, 26, 27, 28, 37, 40, 41, 45,
    75–96, 172, 173
  competency 76–7, 79, 80–5
  nurses' role 91–2
Christensen, P. 11, 26, 35, 37, 43
Chronic Fatigue Syndrome (CFS) 137
chronic condition/illnesses 28, 86, 125, 126, 127,
    128, 129, 135, 137, 138
codes of practice 153–4
cognitive development 81, 123–4
cognitive impairment 2, 102, 124, 139
collaborative participation 44
comfort 1, 61, 99, 105, 106, 112, 114, 115, 139,
    163, 166, 186
communication 2, 9, 11, 22, 40, 45, 47, 54, 58,
    59, 60, 82, 90, 91, 103, 124, 160, 165
community care 100
community nursing, research 47
comparison 1, 5, 137
competency 25, 26, 28, 35, 42, 45, 55, 65, 75,
    76–7, 79, 81, 82, 83, 92, 106, 123, 172
  age 79
  characteristics 80–5
  Gillick competence 79
complaints 155
complex needs 18–19, 47, 127–9
consent, research 80
consultations, information sharing 58–61
consultative participation 44
consulting children 53–74, 154
consumerism 154
continence 75–6, 89
cosmetic procedures 84
Cowley, S. 20, 21
Coyne, I. 20, 21, 47, 78, 89, 123, 125, 130, 132
Crisp, J. 80, 81, 82, 123
critical thinking approach 5
culture 115
  information sharing 60
cystic fibrosis 135

Darvill, J. 105, 128
death 135
  cancer 126, 127
  communication 60
decision making 6, 15, 17, 22, 24, 26, 27, 29, 35,
    39, 40, 41, 44, 45, 75–96, 103, 110, 111, 112,
    151, 164, 165, 172, 173 30–40, 41, 75–96
  competency 76–7, 79, 80–5
  nurses' role 91–2

demographic changes 37
diabetes 6, 9–10, 17–18, 37, 82, 86, 125, 128
Dickinson, A. 108, 156, 165
diet 10, 37
Diffusion of Innovations model 160
disadvantaged children 2, 172
disabled children
  decision making 91
  treatment participation 40
dissent 45, 89–90
Doug, M. 28
Doyon, T. 89
Dozier, M. 102–3

Earle, R. J. 105, 106
early adopters 160–1
Early Support Services Initiative 57
economics 11
Education Act 1870 36
Edwards, M. 123, 125, 128, 130–2, 133, 135–6
Elander, G. 41, 86, 88, 90, 92
Ellison, S. 77, 79, 84
emotional experience and needs 11, 13, 14, 17,
    20, 21, 36, 37, 47, 57, 60, 84, 129, 132
  cancer 127
encopresis 63
environment, best practice 165
epilepsy 136
ethical 22, 33, 43, 44, 45, 60, 114, 115
ethics, research participation 43, 44–5
European Association for Children in Hospital
    (EACH) 16
European Charter for Children in Hospital 16
evaluation 156
Every Child Matters 81
everyday care, decisions 88–9
Evidence Based Nursing (EBN) 151–4
Evidence Based Practice (EBP) 151, 153, 157–8,
    163, 164
exercise 37
existential fear 136–7
experience of illness
  children and young people's 121–48
  competency 80, 81–2

FAME levels 151–2
family
  dynamics 82–5
  hospital visits 11, 13
  nursing proximity 107–8
  space 110
  see also parents
family-centred care 9–10, 16–24, 25
fatigue 129, 134, 136, 137

fear 14, 18, 39, 41, 55, 64, 66, 78, 122, 123, 124,
    127, 127, 130, 132, 133, 135, 136–7, 138, 165
financial costs, FCC 21
focus groups 46, 47
Force Field Analysis 158
Ford, K. 11, 16, 20, 25, 26, 39, 43, 45, 46, 67,
    89, 130, 132–3
Forinder, U. 127, 135
Forsner, M. 122, 124, 125
Franck, L. S. 63–4, 132, 138
Frederiksen, K. 20

games-based methods 46
Garden, 44, 45
Garling Report 14
Gibson, F. 60, 61, 134, 137
Gillick competence 79
Gilmour, J. A. 110–11
Glanz, K. 161
graffiti boards 46
Gray, N. J. 63–4
Greig, A. 36
Gruendel, J. 65
guidelines 163

Hallström, I. 41, 86, 88, 90, 92
Hart, R. 43–4
health consumerism 154
Heaton, J. 100, 105, 106
Hedstrom, M. 127, 133, 135, 136
Hill, M. 11, 45
historical perspective
    of children's health care 11–15
    of children in society 36–7
Hodgkin's lymphoma 33–4
holding children 78, 90
home care 99–100, 113, 172
    technology 105–7
*Hospital: A Deprived Environment for
    Children?* 129
hospitalisation 99, 100–1
    children and adult co-location 27–8
    defining the space 113–17
    experience 129–37
    home like 110–11, 112
    impacts 20
    oral health 149–50, 153, 156, 159, 160, 161–2
Hospital in the Park 101
Huang, I. C. 105–6

information 53–73
    gaining and sharing 20, 54–64, 69, 124
    individual preferences 68, 69
    multiple conditions 57

information *cont.*
    withholding 55–6, 69, 78, 124
injections 18, 53, 67, 123–4, 132–3, 136
Institute for Patient- and Family-Centred Care 20
institutionalisation 102
intensive care 2, 10, 21, 130–2, 163
intergenerational relationships 11
International Children's Palliative Care Network
    (ICPCN) 126
internet
    information 62–4
    online resources 20
    remote care 103–4

Jaaniste, T. 64, 66, 67, 68
James, A. 26, 35, 43, 55, 78, 123
Joanne Briggs Institute (JBI) 152
Joshi, A. 11, 28, 37

Kellett, M. 35, 39, 46
Kennedy, I. 14
key stakeholders 159
Kortesluoma, R. L. 132–3, 137, 138
Kreicbergs, U. 57
Kuo, D. 11, 13, 17, 20, 21

Ladder of Children's Participation 43–4
landscapes of care 98–117
language
    information sharing 60
    treatment participation 40
Lansdown, G. 35, 42, 122
Lansdown, J. 36, 39, 44
leadership 164
    plan for change 159
Leahey, M. 24
legal influence, spaces and places 115–17
Levetown, M. 54–5, 60
Levinson, W. 77
Lewins Force Field Analysis 158
life-course approach 173
life-limiting illnesses/conditions 18, 57, 77, 129
life-world(s) 3, 35, 42
listening to children 39, 43
Locke, J. 36
long-term conditions 57
    competency 81–2
    decision making 86–7
    home care 99
    'right' choice 85

MacDonald, H. 129
MacDonald, M. 21
McLean, C. 157, 159, 161

McMullen, A. 123
Madden, S. 43
Magnet® hospitals 164
maintaining family space 110–11
Malone, R. E. 107–8
Marchionni, C. 153, 159, 162
marginalisation 58, 85
medical error reporting 155
medicalisation 106, 129
mental health problems 40
methylphenidate 47
Mikkelsen, G. 20
Milligan, C. 99, 108
Milnes, L. 59, 85
Mines Act 1842 36
Mirfin-Veitch, B. 103
Moon, G. 98
Moore, A. J. 105, 106, 107, 111, 129
moral proximity 107
Moules, T. 122–3, 138, 139

narrative proximity 107
National Institute for Clinical Excellence (NICE),
    ADHD 46–7
National Service Framework 60
NAWCH 20
needle phobia see injections
Nelson, K. 65
New Zealand Nurses Organisation 4, 7
Nikkonen, M. 132–3, 137, 138
Noble, G. 63–4
normalcy 127, 128

obesity 37, 172
Oldenburg, B. 161
online resources 20
oral health 149–50, 153, 156, 159, 160, 161–2
outcomes 5, 17, 38, 41, 44, 47, 54, 55, 65, 69,
    150, 152, 159, 162, 163, 164, 165, 171,
    172, 173

pain 7, 14, 20, 53, 65, 75, 77, 90, 123, 125, 129,
    132–3, 135, 136, 137–9, 140, 173
parents
  advocacy groups 154
  consultations 58
  decision making 77–8
  hospital participation 21
  information 54–5
  information sharing 60, 69
  presence 13, 16, 21, 130
      hospital visiting 13, 130
  presence and competency 82–5
  terminal illness 57

parents cont.
  timing of information 67
  withholding information 55–6, 69
participation 21, 26, 39–40, 43, 44, 124
  in research 42, 43, 44, 45, 46, 47
partnership approach 24–25, 84
paternalistic model 84
Pearson, A. 151
Paediatric Early Warning Score (PEWS) 163
peer interaction 86, 106
peer pressure 134
'persistent ambivalence' 106
physical appearance 134, 136
physical experience, cancer 127
physical proximity 107
Piaget, J. 81, 123–4
places and spaces 97–120
plan for change 159–60
Platt Report 19
playtime 37
poverty 38
power differentials 45–6, 165
power relations 45
practice development 4, 23, 25, 149, 160, 164, 165
  exercise 22–3
pre-operative/for preparation 65, 133
preparation, procedures, interventions, condition
    changes 64–9, 133
prevalence of illness 122
Pritchard Kennedy, A. 25
privacy 110–11, 113–14
promote/promoting 1, 4, 6, 7, 16, 28, 39, 41, 55,
    77, 78, 91, 92, 122, 150, 161, 162,
    173, 174
Prout, A. 11, 37, 55, 78
proximity 107–8
punishment 130

quality audits 156
quality care 3, 15, 150, 158, 159, 162, 166, 186
quality management 164

Ramsay, J. 122–3, 138, 139
Randhawa, S. 163
Randomised Control Trials (RCT) 151
regime management 86
regulatory influence, spaces and places 115–17
remote care 103–4
renal disease 43
research
  child-centred 45
      difference to research with adults 46
  consent 80
  decision making 79–80

research *cont.*
  ethics 44–5
  participation 42–7
residential care 101–3
rights (children) 34, 36–7, 41
  see also United Nations Convention on the
      Rights of the Child (UNCRC)
Ritchie, J. 153, 159, 162
Roets, L. 21
Rogers, D. M. 160
Rousseau, J.-J. 36
Runeson, I. 78, 80, 83, 89, 90
Rutishauser, C. 85

Savage, E. 58, 133
Schön, D. 22
schools
  assistive devices 105–6
  information sharing 89
script theory 65–6
'seamless web' 19
self-image 134–5, 136
settings 11, 97–120
shared approach 84–5
Shields, L. 16–17, 20, 21–2
side-effects 55–6
Singh, I. 47
Smith-Stoner, M. 103–4
social experience, cancer 127
social factors, decision making 86
social support, internet 63
society 11
Southall, D. 15, 25, 129
spaces/places of care 6, 21, 98, 99, 101, 104, 107,
      109, 110, 111, 113–117
  Landscapes of care 98, 99, 171
standards 14, 15, 27, 36, 37, 48, 80, 103, 115,
      117, 149, 151, 153, 154, 156, 163,
      165, 166
Stang, A. 11, 28, 37
stem cell transplantation 135
steroid therapy 134
Stewart, J. L. 126–7
Stinson, J. N. 63–4
The Strand Magazine 39
surgery 132–3
surveillance 108–9

technology 37
  at home 105–7
  best practice 166
  chronic illness 128–9

technology *cont.*
  dependent 128, 129
  remote care 103–4
telemedicine 103–4
terminal illness 57
Thomas, M. 163
timing, information sharing 66–7
tipping point 161
tokenism 39, 43–4
tonsillectomy 121, 133
'toolkit for child centred asthma care' 59
toys, research methods 46
transformational leadership 159, 164
transition 9, 28–9, 85
translators 60
triadic relationship 84–5
Trollvik, A. 47, 61

understanding of illness 122
United Nations Children's Fund (UNICEF) 37
United Nations Convention on the Rights of the
      Child (UNCRC) 14–15, 16, 34, 36, 172
  best interests 41, 84
  children's views 55
United Nations General Assembly, children's
      decision making 78

venepuncture 132–3
ventilation devices 106
ventilator dependence 90, 129
visual information 61–2
vulnerability 10, 45

Walker, N. E. 89
Watson, J. B. 36
weakness 45
well-being 1, 6, 9, 13, 14, 17, 33, 37, 38, 48, 100,
      115, 117, 125, 134, 147, 166
Willowbrook Study 44
Wilson, M. E. 129
Wise, B. V. 129
withdrawal of care 84
withdrawn children 90
withholding information 55–6, 69, 78, 124
Woodgate, R. 19, 127, 135
World Health Organization 1, 4
  Child Friendly Healthcare Initiative 15
Wright, L. M. 24
written information 61–2

Yoos, H. L. 123
Young, B. 57